MAMMOGRAPHIES

MAMMOGRAPHIES

The Cultural Discourses of Breast Cancer Narratives

Mary K. DeShazer

THE UNIVERSITY OF MICHIGAN PRESS

Ann Arbor

First paperback conversion 2015
Copyright © by the University of Michigan 2013
All rights reserved

Published in the United States of America by
The University of Michigan Press
Manufactured in the United States of America
⊚ Printed on acid-free paper

2018   2017   2016   2015   5   4   3   2

A CIP catalog record for this book is available from the
British Library.

Library of Congress Cataloging-in-Publication Data

DeShazer, Mary K.
    Mammographies : the cultural discourses of breast cancer
narratives / Mary K. DeShazer.
        pages cm
    Includes bibliographical references and index.
    ISBN 978-0-472-11882-3 (cloth : alk. paper) — ISBN 978-0-
472-02923-5 (e-book)
        1. Breast—Radiography—Cross-cultural studies. 2. Breast—
Imaging—Cross-cultural studies. 3. Ethnicity—Health aspects.
4. Transcultural medical care. I. Title.
    RG493.5.R33D47 2013
    618.1'907572—dc23   2013000021

ISBN 978-0-472-03635-6 (paper : alk. paper)

In memory of my beloved friends
Lynda Hart
Billy McClain
Dolly A. McPherson
Elizabeth Phillips

Acknowledgments

Since I could never have written a book about postmillennial representations of breast cancer without the creative visions of the writers, photographers, and scholars whose work I analyze in *Mammographies*, I must first express my gratitude to them for providing me with inspiration. I am indebted to Wake Forest University for awarding me an R. J. Reynolds Faculty Research Leave in 2008–9, during which I conducted much of my research for this study, and an Archie Grant to visit the Jo Spence Memorial Archive in London in 2011. I am grateful to curator Terry Dennett for his assistance at the archive. My colleagues at Wake Forest have been generous in their support; I especially thank English Department Chair Scott Klein and Associate Chair Dean Franco, Women's and Gender Studies Director Wanda Balzano, Rian Bowie, Anne Boyle, Andrew Ettin, Shannon Gilreath, Claudia Kairoff, Mary Martin Niepold, Gillian Overing, Erica Still, Olga Valbuena, and retired colleagues Nancy Cotton, Bob Shorter, and Eva Rodtwitt. For reading my work-in-progress, special thanks go to Anita Helle at Oregon State University, Catherine Keller at Drew University, Patrick Moran at Princeton University, and my WFU transnational feminist theory group: Sally Barbour, Sandya Hewamanne, Catherine Harnois, Judith Madera, and Alessandra Beasley Von Burg. I also appreciate the kindness of WGS administrative coordinators Linda Mecum and Pat Gardea and English Department administrative coordinators Peggy Barrett and Connie Green.

Many dear friends have been cheering me on for years, and I am grateful to have them in my life: Sarah Lu Bradley, E. J. Essic, Gary Ljungquist, Patti Patridge, Inzer Byers, and Rose Simon in North Carolina; Catherine Paul, Sean Scuras, Susan Hilligoss, Kathie Heinz, Donna Reiss, and Art Young in South Carolina; Sandra and Alan Bryant in Kentucky; Susan Carlson, Jane Mead, Monza Naff, and Sharon Ellison in the Bay Area; Martha Kierstead, Cathy Simard, and Nancy Winbigler in Oregon; and Ana Manzanas and Jesús Benito in Salamanca. My family has provided emotional sustenance as well, and I deeply appreciate my siblings, Kathy DeShazer, Sam DeShazer, and Bettye Grogan; my stepdaughter, Sasha Oberbeck; my daughter-in-spirit, Kim Kessaris; my stepsons, Evan Jacobi and Andrew Jacobi; and my wonderful husband, Martin Jacobi. I thank our niece, Megan Brownell, for sharing her own eloquent cancer blog in 2012. And I remain grateful to my late parents, Marian and Henry DeShazer, for all they gave me.

Hearty thanks are due to LeAnn Fields, my editor at the University of Michigan Press, and to her assistant, Alexa Ducsay, for their assistance with this project. I also appreciate the support of the coeditors of journal issues in which my research was published: Jane E. Schultz and Martha Stoddard Holmes, who edited the "Cancer Stories" special issue of *Literature and Medicine,* and Nadine Ehlers and Shiloh Krupar, who edited "The Body in Breast Cancer" special issue of *Social Semiotics.*

An earlier version of the first chapter of this book, "Postmillennial Breast Cancer Photo-narratives: Technologized Terrain," was published in *Social Semiotics* 22, no. 1 (February 2012): 13–30, and is reprinted by permission of the publisher, Taylor & Francis Ltd., http://www.tand fonline.com. An earlier version of chapter 6, "Cancer Narratives and an Ethics of Commemoration: Susan Sontag, Annie Leibovitz, and David Rieff," was published in *Literature and Medicine* 28, no. 2 (Fall 2009): 215–36, and is reprinted by permission of the publisher, The Johns Hopkins University Press.

Contents

Introduction

Representing Breast Cancer in the Twenty-first Century

> Ovarian surgery was only part of the solution. What about breast
> cancer? . . . We couldn't turn our backs on what we knew. We still
> had our family history, even if it was different from the one we
> thought we knew.
> —AMY BOESKY, *What We Have*

> For these young women, having their portrait taken seems to
> represent their personal victory over this terrifying disease. . . .
> Through these simple pictures, they seem to gain acceptance of
> what has happened to them and the strength to move forward
> with pride.
> —DAVID JAY, The SCAR Project

Narratives that explore women's lived experience of breast cancer and
interrogate its cultural discourses provide the focus of my study, which
offers a critical analysis of postmillennial autobiographical and photographic representations of this life-threatening illness. In the texts under
consideration, memoirists and photo-autobiographers probe the ravages
of a still mystifying disease, confront ambivalently its surgical and pharmaceutical treatments, document the physical and psychological processes of recovery, and memorialize the dead. Breast cancer narratives
published in the United States and Great Britain since 2000 differ from
their twentieth-century counterparts in several noteworthy ways. They
address previously neglected topics such as the links between cancer
and environmental carcinogens, the ethics and efficacy of genetic testing
and prophylactic mastectomy, and the shifting politics of prosthesis and
reconstruction. They question the medical establishment for emphasizing detection rather than prevention, and challenge mainstream cancer
culture for its corporate complicity, pink iconography, upbeat rhetoric,
and privileging of philanthropy over activism. They decenter survivor
discourse by paying elegiac tribute to the often invisible women who die
each year of this disease—to their wounded, suffering bodies and the
loss that they instantiate. As catalysts and sites of public memory, these

illness narratives engage readers and viewers politically, ethically, and aesthetically.

Since the publication of my 2005 study of late twentieth-century literary representations of breast, uterine, and ovarian cancers, *Fractured Borders: Reading Women's Cancer Literature,* I have been considering a constellation of issues related to breast cancer and postmillennial literary and visual cultures. This book departs from my previous study and from other scholarship on illness narratives in its exclusive focus on breast cancer, its analysis of both memoirs and photographic narratives, its attention to collaborative and hybrid narratives, and its emphasis on ecological, queer, genetic, transnational, and anti-pink discourses. I argue that, taken together, postmillennial breast cancer narratives, which I refer to as *mammographies,* constitute a distinctive testimonial and memorial tradition whose aims and representational strategies should circulate alongside other cultural projects of memory such as the AIDS memorial quilt (the Names Project). The term *mammographies* signifies both the technology of imaging by which most Western women learn that they have contracted breast cancer and the documentary imperative that drives their written and visual mappings of the breast cancer experience. In the United States alone more than 225,000 women are diagnosed with invasive breast cancer annually, and nearly 40,000 die of it.[1] Worldwide breast cancer rates are rising rapidly, and current projections posit that ten years from now 70 percent of all breast cancer cases will be in developing countries.[2] The scope and parameters of this disease reveal a global crisis. It is therefore unsurprising that not only awareness campaigns and races for the cure abound but also new artistic forms of recounting trauma, celebrating survival, and memorializing the world's dead or dying mothers, daughters, partners, sisters, and friends.

Not everyone who writes breast cancer memoirs has had this disease. Since the 1990 discovery by geneticist Mary-Claire King of a gene linked to hereditary breast cancer, the isolation of that gene—known as BRCA1—in 1994, and the subsequent identification of the BRCA2 gene in 1995, increasing numbers of high-risk but cancer-free women have written what have come to be known as BRCA or "previvor" narratives.[3] These autobiographies trace the authors' family histories of breast and ovarian cancer, chronicle their decision whether to undergo genetic testing, and explore the emotional and medical impact of inherited cancers.[4] Amy Boesky's *What We Have* typifies such narratives in offering a genealogical account of her family's history of ovarian cancer, her mother's death from metastatic breast cancer, her own and her sisters' dawning realization of their high-risk status, and her eventual decision to undergo first a prophylactic oophorectomy, then a bilateral elective mastectomy, without having undertaken the genetic evaluation that would determine whether she carried the BRCA1 mutation. As the epigraph at the beginning of this chapter indicates, Boesky and her siblings recognize after their mother's agonizing demise that they must confront together "what we knew," even if such knowledge was partial, evolving, and alien. "Women in my family die young," Boesky explains near the beginning of her memoir; "I used to walk up and down the hallway and look over this ill-fated, all-female family tree" (23). By choosing preventive breast and ovarian surgeries, she attempts to disrupt the dominant genealogical narrative: "It would be unthinkable, after all this suffering, not to try our hardest to keep this from happening again" (313). That struggle is ongoing, however, since Boesky and her sisters are the mothers of teenaged daughters not yet fully aware of the implications of their legacy.

The postmillennial turn to collaborative narratives can be illustrated by the work of fashion photographer David Jay, who teamed up in 2010 with nearly one hundred women under thirty-five to document visually the loss of their breast(s) to cancer. The result has been a critically acclaimed photographic exhibition and book entitled *The SCAR Project: Breast Cancer Is Not a Pink Ribbon* and a related documentary film by Patricia Zagarella, *Baring It All.*[5] Jay began this project when a thirty-two-year-old model he had known since she was seventeen contracted breast cancer and underwent a mastectomy; he offered support by photographing her in a respectful, unflinching manner. Having recognized the power of such images to raise awareness, Jay recruited young subjects online through breast cancer advocacy organizations and received over a thousand inquiries. A subject named Emily, whose pregnant, scarred body and meditative face appear on the book and poster covers, explains, "When I heard about the SCAR Project, I wanted to be involved. The idea of sharing my own scars to show how breast cancer has impacted another young woman was very compelling. . . . It was an opportunity for me to stand tall and strong with my scars and redefine my beauty for myself" (Q & A). A second subject, Sylvia, twenty-five, posed for the SCAR Project because "I'd just been diagnosed with breast cancer, I really don't know how long I have, so why not do something that will—not keep me here forever—but when I'm gone, there's a part of me that's still left" (www.huffingtonpost.com).

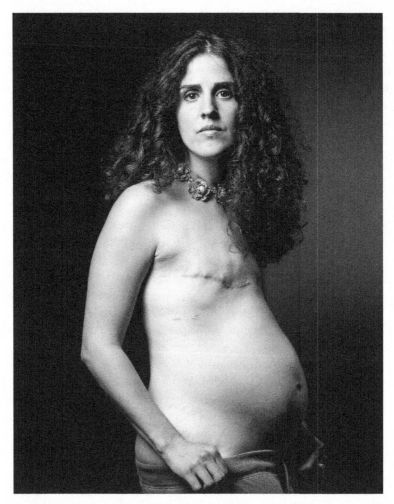

Emily. Courtesy of David Jay, The SCAR Project.

As Jay notes in this introduction's second epigraph, having their vulnerable bodies photographed empowered his subjects, despite the rawness of the images. "I knew in my heart that compromising the visual integrity of the SCAR Project for the sake of easily digested beauty would serve no one," he explains. "Certainly not the people I hoped would be impacted by the images, the public at large who remain blissfully unaware of the risk or reality of this disease anesthetized by pink ribbons and fluffy, pink teddy bears" (McCreery). Although it may be difficult for some viewers to digest, there *is* beauty in Jay's images, as seen in the dig-

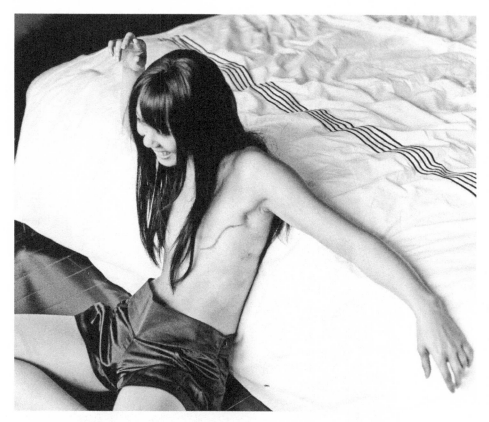

Sylvia. Courtesy of David Jay, The SCAR Project.

nified gaze, luminous face, and muscular one-breasted body of Shanté, who looks pensively at the camera as she bares her mastectomy scar and grasps her belt buckle casually. Projects such as Boesky's and Jay's engage readers and viewers as compassionate witnesses through what scholar Einat Avrahami describes as an implicit contract based on a "reality effect" resulting from intimate narrative revelations that foreground "terminal illness and textually or visually displayed selves" (14–15).

A brief overview of the development of breast cancer narratives as literary and photographic subgenres will help to contextualize the work of Boesky and Jay and to situate my own project historically. As I explained in *Fractured Borders,* memoirs documenting this disease emerged in the United States during the late 1970s and early 1980s as part of the rise of autopathography, life writing about illness. Among the first breast cancer

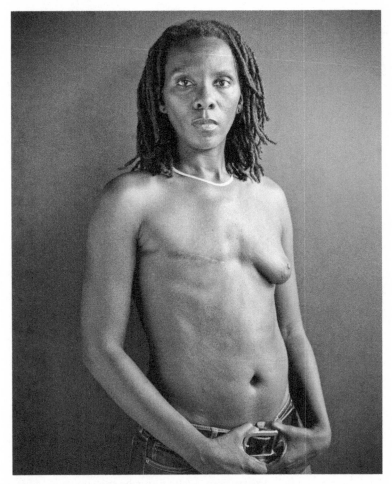

Shanté. Courtesy of David Jay, The SCAR Project.

autobiographies to receive critical attention were activist Rose Kushner's *Breast Cancer: A Personal History and an Investigative Report,* which questioned the ubiquity of the Halsted mastectomy and called for study of environmental causes; journalist Betty Rollin's *First, You Cry,* which brought breast cancer to the attention of mainstream U.S. media; and poet Audre Lorde's *The Cancer Journals,* which offered a Black lesbian feminist account of challenging medical hegemony and eschewing reconstructive surgery. Susan Sontag's 1977 manifesto *Illness as Metaphor* called for a destigmatization of cancer patients and an end to military metaphors of waging war on this disease. During the early 1990s breast cancer memoirs such as Jenny Cole's *Journey (with a Cancer)* and Patricia Duncker's *Cancer: Through the Eyes of Ten Women* were published in England as consciousness-raising works. Analyzing these texts in *Fractured Borders*, I used feminist theory by Elizabeth Grosz and Rosemarie Garland-Thomson to examine five ways in which women's ill bodies were represented—as *medicalized, leaky, amputated, prosthetic, and (not) dying*—and to argue that although cultural stigmatization diminishes ill women's subjectivity, literary depictions of cancer enhance it by providing strategies for resistance, healing, and commemoration. This body of cancer literature grew exponentially throughout the 1990s, as the women's health movement burgeoned, research funding increased dramatically during the Bill Clinton and Tony Blair administrations, and hundreds of writers explored their illness experiences creatively.

Photography also became a public medium for representing breast cancer during the 1980s. A defiant poster featuring a photograph by Hella Hammid that depicted the tattooed mastectomy scar of American poet Deena Metzger circulated widely, as did radical photographs of breasts *Marked Up for Amputation* by British photographer Jo Spence. Like literary representations, photographic depictions of breast cancer flourished in the early 1990s, and a post-mastectomy self-portrait entitled *Beauty Out of Damage* by the one-breasted fashion model Matuschka provoked controversy on the cover of the August 15, 1993, *New York Times Magazine*.[6] Scholar Jean Dykstra correctly notes that while the self-portraits of Matuschka are known for their "polished, fine arts look" and their "pride in a still beautiful body," Spence's photographs offer "in-your-face documentation of her rage and feelings of powerlessness" in the face of this disease (4). Breast cancer photography became more racially diverse during the 1990s as well, when thirty African American women told their cancer stories and posed before the camera lens of Sylvia Dunnavant, who published *Celebrating Life* in 1995 to raise awareness in Black communities. Breast cancer autobiography and photography are thus linked through their publication and reception histories and their narrative strategies of representation. In the twenty-first century increasing numbers of breast cancer memoirs have featured illness photographs and, conversely, photographic narratives have included extensive autobiographical introductions or commentary, making the link between written and visual cancer narratives even stronger.[7]

The shifting contours of breast cancer's discursive and cultural representations are evident when we probe several additional ways in which twenty-first-century narratives differ from their twentieth-century counterparts. One difference is enhanced global awareness. The October 15, 2007, issue of *Time* magazine featured a provocative cover image of a young white woman, torso clothed in a map of the world, intently examining her breast for lumps; its headline reads "Why Breast Cancer Is Spreading Around the World." Inside, an essay by Kathleen Kingsbury noted that 500,000 new and current breast cancer patients around the globe would die that year and offered testimonials from patients in China, India, Kenya, South Africa, Egypt, and elsewhere. The article pointed out that while breast cancer incidences are rising due to Western "meat-sweet" diets, high rates of obesity, immigration patterns, and possible environmental causes, early detection and treatment advances are not keeping pace transnationally. In Kenya, reported Mary Onyango, breast cancer feels hopeless to most women who contract it: "If you can't travel overseas for treatment, you just sit and wait for your death" (Kingsbury, 37). Chinese patient Liu Lichun testified that she had never known about mammograms or mastectomies before contracting breast cancer and connecting with the U.S.-based advocacy group Susan G. Komen for the Cure: "I'd never heard of anyone in China with cancer who didn't die" (Kingsbury, 36). The Lebanese writer Evelyne Accad explains in *The Wounded Breast* that many Arabic-speaking people "refer to cancer as *Al-marad illi ma btitssamma:* the disease not to be named"; she writes her memoir to work against silence and stigmatization in the Middle East (29). In *Manmade Breast Cancers* (2001) U.S. activist Zillah Eisenstein likewise posits a global imperative by developing "a breast-felt politics" and tracing "a theorized journey from my body to a politics of bodies for a healthful globe" (x, 61).

Furthermore, U.S. and British breast cancer narratives have become increasingly multicultural. They feature significant racial-ethnic, religious, sexual, national, and age diversity, a range of voices and images that I have attempted to capture in *Mammographies*. The writers, photographers, and photographic subjects I examine are African American, White, Latina, Asian American, and Native American; Jewish, Muslim, Christian, and secular; Iranian, Lebanese, Canadian, and Dominican as well as American and British; lesbians as well as heterosexuals; old and middle-aged women as well as young; male, female, and transgendered. Such diversity of focus is important not only for feminist inclusivity but also because of differential risk factors and disease outcomes. Ashkenazi

Jews are disproportionately vulnerable to BRCA mutations, for example, while African Americans, Native Americans, and lesbians with breast cancer are more likely to die of it than Caucasians are, for reasons having to do with genetics, childbirth status, economics, and/or treatment access.[8]

Another way that postmillennial writing differs from earlier narratives lies in its critiques of mainstream cancer culture. Taken as a whole, the visual and verbal narratives that make up this study tend to question hegemonic cultural discourses and work against the consumer-oriented breast cancer culture that emerged in the West during the last two decades of the twentieth century—a sentimental culture characterized by the "pink kitsch" of the cancer marketplace (Barbara Ehrenreich's term) and the corporate rallying of "Pink Ribbons, Inc." with its defining "tyranny of cheerfulness" (Samantha King's phrases).[9] In her influential 2010 study *Pink Ribbon Blues* writer-activist Gayle Sulik critiques the corporate-driven development of "pink ribbon culture," examines how mainstream media and breast cancer organizations promote pink products through "conscientious consumerism" and sell "survivorship," and argues for a radical rethinking of this cultural phenomenon. David Jay echoes this critique in his commentary on the SCAR Project's subtitle: "Many women battling breast cancer dislike the pink ribbon. They resent the commercialization of breast cancer that it represents. One of the SCAR Project subjects said to me, 'If a man got prostate cancer, do you think someone would give him a pink t-shirt and teddy bear?' It (unintentionally) diminishes something that is horrific, disfiguring, and deadly. A pink herring" (McCreery). While many breast cancer narrators appreciate the designation of October as National Breast Cancer Awareness Month and honor organizations such as Susan G. Komen for the Cure for its global advocacy, activists such as Ehrenreich, King, Sulik, and Jay challenge the corporate politics and consumerism that such initiatives endorse.

An additional characteristic of postmillennial representations of breast cancer is the rise of new narrative forms, notably graphic narratives and blogs. As Hillary Chute points out in *Graphic Women,* comics constitute an evolving form of "feminist cultural production" that offers "a new aesthetic emerging around self-representation that is both written and drawn" (1). While feminist graphic narratives address themes from sexuality to abuse to childhood memories, an important subset depicts the breast cancer experience, as illustrated by Marisa Acocella Marchetto's *Cancer Vixen,* Miriam Engelberg's *Cancer Made Me a Shallower Person,* and Brian Fies's *Mom's Cancer,* all of which blend wry humor and intimate confession in whimsically drawn portraits of a self in crisis. Breast cancer blogs also abound in postmillennial culture, among them the *Y-me Forums* (www.forums.y-me.org) and Breast Cancer Action's *Think Before You Pink* campaign (www.bcaction.org).

Defiant feminist blogs posted by spirited advocates have also gained cultural capital. Noteworthy examples include the late Rachel Moro's *The Cancer Culture Chronicles* (www.cancerculturenow.blogspot.com), which critiqued pink consumerism as "insane," provided updates on the blogger's struggle with metastatic breast cancer, and garnered hundreds of weekly responses until the author's death in 2012; and Peggy Orenstein's postings (www.peggyorenstein.com/blog) on the inanities of breast cancer consumerism, which feature such titles as "The Trouble with Those Boobie Bracelets." Blogs such as *Komenwatch* (www.komen watch.org) that critique the methodology of Susan G. Komen for the Cure have gained readership, especially in light of the December 2011 controversy over that organization's decision, ultimately retracted, to withdraw funds from Planned Parenthood that paid for underserved women's mammograms.[10] In her 2012 essay "Moving Beyond Pink Ribbons" Orenstein claims that only 15 percent of Komen's budget in 2008 was allocated for research, whereas 55 percent ($200 million) went to "awareness education"—in her mind, a misplaced priority. Gayle Sulik's blog (www.gaylesulik.com) likewise challenges the corporate ties of Susan G. Komen for the Cure; in February 2012 she asked, "Is Komen 'Losing the Brand'?" Feminist graphic narratives and blogs focused on breast cancer often bring critical or humorous lenses to a profoundly serious subject.

A final distinctive feature of twenty-first-century breast cancer narratives is their emphasis on memorialization of nonsurvivors alongside the honoring of people living with this disease. Critiques of the word *survivor* and of mainstream cancer organizations' emphasis on survivorship often arise in contemporary breast cancer narratives. This trend began with Ehrenreich's 2001 essay "Welcome to Cancerland," where she argued powerfully that "the mindless triumphalism of 'survivorhood' denigrates the dead and the dying. Did we who live 'fight' harder than those who have died? Can we claim to be 'braver,' better, people than the dead?" (53). The postmillennial turn to breast cancer autothanatography, life writing about dying, provides a vital cultural counternarrative, as women living with metastatic disease recount their embodied struggles and their fierce resolve to embrace life for as long as they can. As Laura E. Tanner notes in *Lost Bodies,* "Thinking about the body in the context of mortality shakes up our assumptions of the body's transparency" (6). Despite the textual and ethical challenges of "introducing the lost body into the literary image, the photographic frame, the public space," narrative representations of suffering and grief affirm critically ill bodies otherwise "lost to cultural view" (2.5). The increasing publication of end-of-life narratives that contain introductions or conclusions penned by friends and family constitutes an evolving memorial tradition that empowers reader-viewers as empathic witnesses and provides communal spaces for mourning and remembering.

Mammographies engages all of the postmillennial features of breast cancer narratives noted above, along with many others. My scholarly approach—best characterized as literary critical, feminist, and interdisciplinary—includes detailed interpretation of the narrative strategies, thematic contours, and visual imagery in the texts under consideration. I deploy a range of theoretical perspectives including gender studies, photographic history and theory, medical humanities, disability studies, queer theory, and trauma studies. More specifically, I investigate a diverse range of memoirs and photographic narratives and consider what they signify culturally and how they invite audiences to respond. Activist memoirs that theorize the disease from feminist, queer, transnational, and/or environmentalist perspectives call for political action and for a scholarly and cultural emphasis on causes and prevention as well as on awareness and cure. Genealogical memoirs that explore genetic testing and prophylactic mastectomy engage the culturally vexed topic of inherited breast cancer and depict the writers' struggles to make agonizing decisions regarding contingent embodiment, contested knowledge, and familial responsibility. Subversive memoirs that use rebellious humor to represent the breast cancer experience as wryly comic rather than (or as well as) tragic reflect the perspectives of women "living in prognosis" (S. Lochlann Jain's phrase) or approaching death defiantly.[11]

With regard to breast cancer photography, this project explores new trends since the late 1990s, most notably the movement away from individual self-portraiture to collaborative photographic narratives. In terms of shifting visual imagery, I analyze not only photographs of women's scarred, post-operative breasts but also of their lymphedema, the arm swelling that can accompany mastectomy when lymph nodes are removed, and of the hair loss that strikes most recipients of chemotherapy and often leads to preemptive and sometimes communal head-shaving. I interrogate as well raw and controversial photographs of women hospitalized, dying, and dead from breast cancer and explore their ethical and commemorative dimensions. And I move from indexical to iconic representation to explore memorial photographs of what remains: the abandoned running shoes, the unfinished book manuscripts, the shell and stone collections of women dead from cancer: ghostly traces of lives cut short.

In chapter 1, "Postmillennial Breast Cancer Photo-narratives: Technologized Terrain," I use theoretical insights by Sidonie Smith and Julia Watson to consider how tropes of experience, identity, embodiment, agency, and memory circulate in contemporary breast cancer photographic narratives, and I assess what the phrase *technologized terrain* signifies discursively and theoretically. I then analyze the queer theorizing, postmodern rhetoric of indeterminacy, and narrative performance of hair loss that characterize Catherine Lord's 2004 photo-narrative *The Summer of Her Baldness*. I go on to explore photographer Lynn Kohlman's commentary and technologically marked self-portraits in *Lynn Front to Back* (2005), the photo-narrative she published during her struggle with breast and brain cancer. In closing I discuss the ethical capacities of postmillennial breast cancer narratives and use critical arguments by philosophers Sara Ahmed and Kelly Oliver to gesture toward issues of witness and memorialization that I develop in subsequent sections of this study.

The next three chapters investigate the cultural discourses that inform contemporary memoirs written by women confronting breast cancer. In chapter 2, "Audre Lorde's Successors: Breast Cancer Narratives as Feminist Theory," I probe the narrative strategies of theorists who employ feminist and ecological consciousness in hybrid texts that serve simultaneously as illness memoirs and environmental polemics. These writers extend the pioneering scholarship of Lorde, who in *The Cancer Journals* (1980) and *A Burst of Light* (1988) presented the perspective of a "Black lesbian feminist warrior poet" and made visible the gendered, racial, and capitalist politics of this disease. I argue that Zillah Eisenstein's *Manmade Breast Cancers* (2001), Evelyne Accad's *The Wounded Breast: Intimate Journeys Through Cancer* (2001), and three essays published between 2007 and 2010 by S. Lochlann Jain—"Cancer Butch," "Living in Prognosis," and "Be Prepared"—extend Lorde's feminist critique by interrogating the Western medical establishment's corporate ties and narrow range of cancer treatment protocols. These narratives further assert links between environmental carcinogens and the worldwide rise in breast cancer, challenge U.S. cancer culture for its emphasis on survivorship and hyperfemininity, and decry racist and heterosexist assumptions regarding global women's cancer risks, experiences, and prognoses.

Chapter 3, "Narratives of Prophylactic Mastectomy: Mapping the Breast Cancer Gene," examines memoirs from England and the United States that chronicle inherited breast cancer and women's decisions to undergo preventive mastectomies in hopes of avoiding the fate of grandmothers, mothers, and/or sisters who died of the disease. Since researchers identified the BRCA1 gene in 1994 and BRCA2 in 1995, writers with a genetic predisposition toward breast cancer have begun to publish genealogical narratives. Among them are Janet Reibstein's *Staying Alive: A Family Memoir* (2002), Elizabeth Bryan's *Singing the Life: A Family in the Shadow of Cancer* (2007), and Jessica Queller's *Pretty Is What Changes: Impossible Choices, the Breast Cancer Gene, and How I Defied My Destiny* (2008). I argue that these prophylactic mastectomy narratives feature pedagogical, memorializing, and autobiographical imperatives, and I assess their cultural and aesthetic impact as well as their shortcomings, notably the writers' tendency toward a "single causality" approach to breast cancer, their lack of environmental consideration, and their (perhaps inevitable) use of competing discourses of biological determinism and self-determination.

Chapter 4, "Rebellious Humor in Breast Cancer Narratives: Deflating the Culture of Optimism," focuses on narratives that employ incongruity, wit, and anti-pink humor as subversive antidotes to the terror and despair that often accompany breast cancer diagnoses and treatments. "Humor is not resigned, it is rebellious," claimed Freud, and memoirists who scoff at breast cancer culture and evoke their readers' empathic laughter agree. Meredith Norton's *Lopsided: How Having Breast Cancer Can Be Really Distracting* (2008), Miriam Engelberg's *Cancer Made Me a Shallower Person* (2006), and S. L. Wisenberg's *The Adventures of Cancer Bitch* (2009) use ironic self-deprecation, tropes of self-division, and strategic self-assertion to defy breast cancer and the cancer marketplace as well as to confront their fears of debilitation and premature death. I argue that, paradoxically, the comic self-scrutiny and transgressive humor of these memoirs undermine the tyrannical cheerfulness that Samantha King rightly identifies as widespread in twenty-first-century breast cancer culture. In addition, I use Jo Anna Isaak's theories of strategic narcissism and Hillary Chute's insights into feminist graphic narratives to analyze the aesthetic impact and cultural critique that underlie the narrative form that each humorist chooses, from Norton's hilarious pseudoconfessional mode to Engelberg's sequential "memoir in comics" to Wisenberg's combative, blog-centered text.

The next two chapters concentrate on shifting postmillennial trends in photographic representations of breast cancer. In chapter 5, "New Directions in Breast Cancer Photography: Documenting Women's Postoperative Bodies," I trace briefly the late twentieth-century history of cancer self-portraiture, then explore the turn toward collaborative photonarratives. Disconcerting images of women's breasts after lumpectomy or mastectomy, defiant or depleted bodies, and bald heads following chemotherapy drive the five collections under consideration: Art Myers's *Winged Victory: Altered Images Transcending Breast Cancer* (1996), Amelia Davis's *The First Look* (2000), Jila Nikpay's *Heroines: Transformation in the Face of Breast Cancer* (2006), Amy S. Blackburn and Cynthia Ogden's *Caring for Cynthia* (2008), and Charlee Brodsky and Stephanie Byram's *Knowing Stephanie* (2003). Issues of visual rhetoric and representation with which I grapple include concealment versus revelation of post-surgical bodies, cultural fetishizing of healthy breasts and stigmatizing of "debreasted" embodiment, the cultural and emotional stakes of representing mastectomy scars (whether bare or tattooed), photographic challenges to hegemonic definitions of beauty and femininity, and visual strategies of eulogizing. I share scholar Lisa Cartwright's view that mainstream media feature as breast cancer's iconic "survivors" women who are young, white, thin, and glamorous. In analyzing what breast cancer does and means in contemporary Western cultures I thus consider not only *how* women's post-surgical bodies are documented but also *whose* bodies are represented, and why. Building on Ehrenreich's critique of breast cancer culture, I discuss ambivalent photo-narrative discourses of transcendence and triumphalism as well as liberating feminist discourses of self-disclosure and collaboration.

In chapter 6, "Cancer Narratives and an Ethics of Commemoration: Susan Sontag, Annie Leibovitz, and David Rieff," I consider how different forms of photographic and biographical memorialization pay tribute to women who die from cancer, inviting reader-viewers to respond with empathy rather than voyeurism. My argument pivots on the controversial photographs by Leibovitz in *A Photographer's Life* (2006) of Sontag during her decades-long struggle with cancer—from mastectomy to chemotherapy to bone marrow transplant to decline and death—and on the memoir of his mother's final year by Sontag's son, David Rieff, *Swimming in a Sea of Death* (2008). Drawing on analyses of trauma and visual representation by art historians Bracha L. Ettinger and Griselda Pollock, I argue that both Leibovitz's nonsequential photographic narrative and Rieff's biographical narrative offer grim, disturbing, yet eloquent and ultimately ethical commemorations of Sontag's painful death from cancer and that by extension they help reader-viewers bear witness to and mourn the cancer deaths of others.

Chapter 7, "Bodies, Witness, Mourning: Reading Breast Cancer Autothanatography," uses Susanna Egan's theories from *Mirror Talk* and Sidonie Smith's theories from "Identity's Body" to scrutinize this chapter's focal conceptual framework: life writing about dying. As case studies I contrast the narrative strategies of two journalistic autothanatographies, one premillennial and the other postmillennial: Ruth Picardie's *Before I Say Goodbye: Recollections and Observations from One Woman's Final Year* (1997) and Dina Rabinovitch's *Take Off Your Party Dress: When Life's Too Busy for Breast Cancer* (2007). Both women were British journalists who wrote widely acclaimed feature columns (and in Rabinovitch's case, a popular blog) about their experience of living with and dying of breast cancer, Picardie in 1997 in *Observer Life* and Rabinovitch from 2004 to 2007 in the *Guardian*. Although each memoirist employs maternal, medicalized, and sartorial discourses to parse her cancer story publicly, Picardie's twentieth-century narrative offers no cultural critique, while Rabinovitch's twenty-first-century narrative uses a rhetoric of outrage to question medical experimentation, the economics of breast cancer, and the ubiquitous pinkwashing of the cancer marketplace. As autothanatographers, both Picardie and Rabinovitch display maternal anguish and instantiate self-memorialization, and like Leibovitz and Rieff, they engage readers as empathic witnesses. To conclude this chapter I apply concepts of communal grief and grievability articulated by Judith Butler to the project of breast cancer autothanatography.

Finally, in "Afterword: What Remains," I examine unsettling photographic traces of the lives of three writers in this study cut short by untimely deaths from cancer. I consider the indexical and iconographic significance of Stephanie Byram's running shoes, worn in several cancer marathons and captured photographically by Charlee Brodsky; Dina Rabinovitch's jaunty chapeau, depicted in the final posting of her blog, "Take Off Your Running Shoes" and described as the perfect hat for a woman wheelchair-bound and balding at forty-four; and Susan Sontag's incomplete manuscripts, shell collection, and empty Manhattan apartment window as captured in memorial photographs by Annie Leibovitz. I explore what reader-viewers might make of these photographs—emotionally, ethically, and aesthetically—and engage scholar Marianne Hirsch's concept of "enlarging the postmemorial circle" as a site of grief and remembrance.

Mammographies extends feminist knowledge of breast cancer by examining a wide array of postmillennial visual and verbal narratives and situating them culturally, discursively, and sociohistorically. My hope is that professors and students of literature, medical humanities, gender studies, and the visual arts, along with medical practitioners and health care professionals, will find this study useful. I write especially to honor breast cancer patients, former patients, and activists, as well as the friends and families of women and men who did not survive this disease.

1 | Postmillennial Breast Cancer Photo-narratives
Technologized Terrain

Visual and autobiographical narratives that explore women's lived experience of breast cancer and its cultural discourses are the subject of this book, which offers a critical analysis of postmillennial representations of a gendered and potentially lethal illness.[1] I call such narratives *mammographies,* a term that signifies both the technology of imaging by which most Western women learn that they have contracted this disease and the documentary imperatives that drive their written and visual mappings of the "breast cancer continuum" (King, xviii).[2] Photographic narratives that interrogate breast cancer's material and technologized terrain provide this chapter's focus, as I consider the representational dynamic between image and text in postmodern life-writing in which self-portraiture and medicalization feature prominently. As Paul Jay notes in "Posing: Autobiography and the Subject of Photography," visual memory plays as central a role as historical memory in memoirs that feature "both the photograph as a subject *in* autobiography, and the subject as he or she comes to be defined by a photograph reproduced (or alluded to) in an autobiography" (191).[3] The visual terrain that breast cancer photo-narratives map evokes different registers of the term *technologized:* photography as a technology, photographs as a means of documenting the technologies of breast cancer treatment, the photographic representation of technological imaging in/as a diagnostic or medical protocol, and the ways in which ill and medicalized bodies are mediated by technology.[4] To examine ways in which narrators and reader-viewers of breast cancer photo-narratives construct multiple meanings regarding the somatic and symbolic contours of this disease, I address issues of contingent embodiment, visual/verbal representation, and viewer/reader reception, and I explore these questions: What distinctive contributions to readers' and viewers' understandings of women's material and technologized bodies do breast cancer photo-narratives offer? How might feminist theories of illness, autobiography, and embodiment, and postmodern constructions of narrative subjectivity, enhance analysis and interpretation of breast cancer's textual and visual representations? What tropes and personae, visual and rhetorical strategies, ethical and aesthetic debates, and opportunities for discursive resistance and/or audience witness do such narratives engage?

As Sidonie Smith and Julia Watson note in their introduction to *Interfaces: Women/Autobiography/Image/Performance*, "telling is performative; it enacts the 'self' that it claims has given rise to an 'I.' And that 'I' is neither unified nor stable—it is fragmented, provisional, multiple, in process" (9). Nowhere are these postmodern axioms of performativity and contingency more apparent than in breast cancer photo-narratives, which render the complex subjectivities of women struggling to come to terms with a frightening and disruptive medical diagnosis, invasive surgery (usually lumpectomy or mastectomy), subsequent debilitating treatments such as chemotherapy and/or radiation, and shifting, often speculative prognoses that might indicate either remission or metastasis but rarely guarantee freedom from cancer, let alone cure. As Smith and Watson further note, "autobiographical acts of narration, situated in historical time and cultural place, deploy discourses of identity to organize acts of remembering that are directed to multiple addressees or readers. . . . They are performative, situated addresses that invite their readers' collaboration in producing specific meanings for the 'life'" (11).

In *Reading Autobiography*, Smith and Watson offer a useful theoretical model for analyzing contemporary breast cancer memoirs by identifying five key "constitutive processes of autobiographical subjectivity": identity, experience, embodiment, agency, and memory (15–16). The identity that the narrator of a breast cancer photo-narrative constructs engages a speaking or a visually rendered "self" at once discursive and provisional, intersectional and unfixed. The lived experience that an autobiographer seeks to describe initiates a process of identity formation that involves interactions with material, cultural, economic, and psychic forces; these interactions, in turn, give rise to various forms of somatic and narrative subjectivity. Embodiment as a critical concept acknowledges bodies as sites of autobiographical knowledge, and narrators as anatomically, genetically, imaginatively, and sociopolitically situated. A struggle to claim some form of agency in the face of breast cancer's somatic and technologized terrain informs the narrating subject's methods of self-representation, whether utilizing shifting narrative strategies, negotiating cultural constrictions, or envisioning multiple or contingent forms of embodiment. Memory serves breast cancer photo-autobiographers as a tool for creating meaning from an unrecoverable past by organizing material experience into narrative and visual testimony that moves, illuminates, or unsettles viewer-readers, who in turn collaborate (actively or implicitly) in acts of witness and spectatorship. Smith and Watson summarize well the autobiographical imperatives that inform postmillennial breast cancer photo-narratives: "As a moving target, a set of shifting self-referential practices, autobiographical narration offers occasions for negotiating the past, reflecting on identity, and critiquing cultural norms and narratives" ("Introduction," *Interfaces,* 8–9).

In *The Invading Body: Reading Illness Autobiographies* Einat Avrahami argues that contemporary illness narratives "underline the uneasy coexistence of the lived body with the multiply inscribed cultural body" and compel an implicit reader-viewer-writer-photographer contract based on a "reality effect" that she defines as a connection established through narrative revelation of a traumatized self-in-crisis (8, 14). Discussing the "contingent and contiguous relationships between writers' and artists' experience of [potentially] terminal illness and their textually or visually displayed selves," Avrahami suggests that illness photo-narratives comprise "an emerging subgenre of self-documentation whose indexical relationship with the reality of illness parallels the contiguity of [nonvisual] illness narratives with somatic experience" (3, 19). Avrahami builds on work of earlier scholars of autopathography (life writing about illness), notably G. Thomas Couser, who has theorized representations of recovering and vulnerable bodies in illness autobiographies; Arthur Frank, who has theorized the liberatory and delimiting dimensions of illness restitution narratives; and Leigh Gilmore, who has theorized the relationship among narrative subjectivity, the material body, and somatic memory by raising such compelling questions as "What does skin have to do with autobiography?" and "What sort of muse, guide, or judge is memory?" (15).[5] In examining affinities between autobiographical and photographic representations of illness, Avrahami extends the scope of earlier theorists and anticipates this study's parameters.

As a distinctive subset of illness narratives, postmillennial breast cancer photo-narratives reflect complex issues of subjectivity, embodiment, and medical prognosis. Many writers and photographers represent their cancer experience from a retrospective vantage point; such narratives may follow a linear, restitutive trajectory—from diagnosis to treatment to a tentative, contingent recovery—or they may offer circular, fragmented, or multimedia structures that include journal entries, emails, poems, photographic collages, or "then versus now" temporal juxtapositions. These narrators recount verbally and visually their surgical/technological/pharmaceutical treatments and their subsequent suffering and/or rehabilitation, and they simultaneously critique hegemonic cultural discourses about the breast cancer body. Some writer-photographers move from autopathography to autothanatography, a focus that juxtaposes the somatic and technologized experience of breast cancer to the patient's recurrence and decline. In that case reader-viewers may undertake a particularly daunting and ethically fraught task of witness. Although autothanatography might initially seem to be a subgenre of illness narratives, *all* memoirs and photographs are haunted by mortality. Susanna Egan, a feminist theorist of autothanatography, makes this point in *Mirror Talk: Genres of Crisis in Contemporary Autobiography:* "The spectre of death hovers over all autobiography, usually unnamed, providing serious impetus to the activity of setting the record straight, clearing old scores, avoiding misinterpretation, taking control of the absolutely uncontrollable— the 'end of the story'" (196). In *On Photography* Susan Sontag makes a similar claim: "Photographs state the innocence, the vulnerability of lives heading toward their own destruction and this link between photography and death haunts all photographs of all people." For this reason, she concludes, "all photographs are *memento mori*" (3–4).

A close analysis of Catherine Lord's *The Summer of Her Baldness* (2004) and Lynn Kohlman's *Lynn Front to Back* (2005) will illuminate the shifting representational terrain of breast cancer photo-narratives. The politics of location and narrative subjectivities of these two autobiographers differ. Lord, a lesbian feminist artist and photographer born on the Caribbean island of Dominica and now residing in the United States, was in her early fifties, living with a long-term partner, and writing a book on Dominica when diagnosed with stage-two breast cancer with lymph node involvement in May 2000. Shortly after her diagnosis she postponed her research and adopted the email-centered nom de plume Her Baldness as a wry voice through whom to inform friends and family of her cancer and treatment protocol: lumpectomy followed by six to nine months of chemotherapy and radiation. Using this wry doppelganger as a way "to make illness a space of language," Lord subsequently converted her emails and documentary photographs into a queer feminist photo-narrative subtitled *A Cancer Improvisation* (237). Kohlman, a world-renowned American fashion model whose airbrushed image appeared on the covers of *Vogue, Elle,* and *Harper's Bazaar* throughout the 1970s, spent subsequent decades as an advertising designer for Anne Klein and DKNY before being diagnosed in 2002 with stage-three breast cancer, in 2003 with stage-four brain cancer. She was in her fifties, married with a teenage son, and a professional photographer at the time of her cancer diagnoses, which she later described as terrifying: "The first time, in September 2002, it was my right breast, and I was emotionally numb. The second time, in October 2002, it was my left breast, and I was devastated. The third time, in March 2003, it was my brain, and I felt like I was falling into an unimaginable, endless black abyss" (np). Kohlman underwent a double mastectomy followed months later by brain surgery; both procedures necessitated extensive radiation and chemotherapy, after which she determined to break silence about her illnesses by publishing a photo-narrative driven by discourses of somatic defiance and spiritual healing despite her dire prognosis. Kohlman's discursive position is thus implicitly autothanatographic, whereas Lord's narrative stance tends toward autopathography and restitution.

Despite these salient differences, Lord and Kohlman employ similar textual strategies to inscribe invasive medicalization and somatic and discursive resistance. As we shall see, they present compelling self-portraiture and high-tech visual imagery of their breast cancer bodies as central to their narratives, and they invite reader-viewers to engage with them as empathic witnesses.

Performing Butch Baldness:
Catherine Lord's Photo-narrative

Catherine Lord's photographic memoir, *The Summer of Her Baldness,* addresses an email listserv known as "FOCL'SRB" (Friends of Catherine Lord's Right Breast), chronicles her treatment for invasive breast cancer from May 2000 to February 2001, and introduces reader-viewers to Her Baldness, the persona Lord adopts while documenting her illness via writing and photographs. As reviewer Delease Wear notes, "The most intriguing aspect of this improvisation is Her Baldness, a quick-tempered, passionate presence who 'talks big' and 'talks a lot,'" yet this seductive and sometimes annoying amanuensis "is more than Lord's witty experiment in narration. She is also an enactment of the fluidity of identity, here the 'conflicted relationship' between the before-she-got-breastcancer-Catherine Lord and the postdiagnosis, bald, bolder, uncensored Catherine Lord" (Wear, 378). The centrality of the trope of self-division to Lord's narrative is evident from Wear's analysis; Lord further exploits that trope by framing the dated chapters of her image text with a prologue and an epilogue, written retrospectively, that blur the distinction between writer and persona. Threaded among the sections of her verbal narrative, usually by way of introducing chapters, are self-portraits of her bald pate and photographs of the mammography machines, breast scans, and hospital warning signs that document her lived experience of medicalization.

Lord's narrative is informed by feminist, queer, and postmodern theories of gender, sexuality, illness, and embodiment. Early on she admits uncomfortably that she dreads going bald more than facing lumpectomy or chemotherapy; subsequent emails thus present her responses to alopecia, from embarrassment to grief to theorization.[6] Lord positions hair presence and absence as a queer feminist issue and a culturally inflected symbol of gender identity. "Looking Backward," the narrative's prologue, orients reader-viewers by explaining that Her Baldness (subsequently HB) first appeared on "the day my hair lost the last battle," this persona having decided to "launch herself into the void like Yves Klein (who, after all, faked the photograph) or Thelma and Louise (who couldn't be allowed to live in America) or the postqueer hacker cyber assassin I wish I were (although that woman is younger, hasn't caught cancer yet, and has more energy than I do) . . ." (5). Here Lord combines strategic self-deprecation with wry references to renegade figures from popular visual culture; her allusion to the "postqueer" cyberhacker reveals as well an affinity for postmodern feminist underground humor. Lord's subsequent assessment of HB reveals both self-judgment and grudging gratitude. On the one hand HB "had her petty moments": she could be manipulative, whiny, and vindictive; she was often misguided and still more often frightened; and she not only had "caught cancer but she had contracted the two most common symptoms of cancer: Unwanted Aloneness and Loss of Control. Instead of being angry at her cancer, or the idea of cancer, or evolution . . . or advanced capitalism, she got mad at people she knew," excising them from her listserv when their responses failed to please her (3). In short, Lord insists retrospectively, HB was a wimp, an autocrat, and a poseur.

On the other hand, as an avenging doppelganger HB provides Lord with a fiercely resistant voice and the zany nerve of a striptease artist.

> Her Baldness . . . made up this list so that she could be strong and
> proud and brave and full of energy and motion in the middle of
> the desolation that is cyberspace, even if she hated how she looked
> and it took pretty much all she had sometimes to get down the
> stairs to the computer in her studio and stay there. . . . She plucked
> an audience out of thin air. Having done so, she played it shame-
> lessly. She sang for her supper. She danced for her dinner. She
> stripped for sympathy. She posted her fear. (3–4)

The rhetorical strategy of parallelism invests this passage with an incan-
tatory rhythm, while the catalog of HB's rebellious performative gestures
and reliance on a loyal if voyeuristic audience provides both psychological confession and jolting humor. Lord thus juxtaposes ironic self-
deprecation and liberating self-assertion to ascribe to HB a transgressive
agency and an authoritative voice that both verbalizes and deflects Lord's
fears of cancer, medicalization, and mortality.

Lord's queer positionality offers her a lens through which to depict her
cancer experience as discursive, postmodern, and transgendered. Early
in her narrative she politicizes breast cancer by comparing her email revelations to coming-out: "It's like coming out of the closet. You don't do
it just once, and once you've done it you can never stop. . . . Cancer is a
disease I can't just have, or be . . . but an identity I must state, or choose
not to state, at every encounter" (18). To seize discursive and imaginative
control over her disease, she uses language as a means of reconceptual-
izing her gender identity: "*Remember, speculate, invent, get it down, make
language fly, whirl in my own baldness. My world, my language, my mind.
A new gender*" (18). Hairlessness transforms her from femme to butch,
she later notes, but accepting baldness is nonetheless difficult. Although
Lord is initially proud of the "outrageously mannish invert butchly LES-
BIAN haircut" that her hair loss from chemo necessitates, she quickly
recognizes its stigmatizing aspects: "*Metastatic art world gossip. I am being recategorized from invincible castrating lesbian bitch to has-been on
her last legs. She used to be so tough. That's what they'll say. She must have
gone downhill*" (32). Nonetheless, Lord determines to deflect the stare
of others—that objectifying gaze that, as Rosemarie Garland-Thomson
has shown, is used to mark bodily differences as deviant (*Staring*, 1–5).
Instead of confronting the starers verbally, Lord resolves simply to "*Be
bald. Take it as a badge of honor,*" since she recognizes that despite her
illness she still can write, laugh, and take disparagement in stride: "The

performance performs the performer. If you don't let bald in, neither can other people. . . . Collect the stares and use them later" (33, 40). Yet the fact remains that hair loss unsettles Her Baldness. As "a signifier that has detached itself from its time," Lord notes, "my hair [is] dead, a museum of female insecurity and lesbian codes" (35).

Despite these concerns, hair loss ultimately provides Lord with a touchstone for theorizing gender, culture, power.

> Hair is something the strong strip from the weak, be they animals or wayward women or boot camp recruits. My skull felt thinner, as if it could crack wide open in a social setting, and the mirror in a middle-aged woman's bathroom is not a private place. It is irrevocably and inexorably a social setting. (36)

Once the narrator verbalizes her hair loss anxiety to her "queer family" via email, she employs HB to reimagine baldness as strength—at once a location from which to interrogate public-private binaries, an aesthetic preference to affirm, and a defiant political stance against the thralldom of hegemonic femininity. Ultimately the narrator refuses to wear a wig but instead embraces her shiny pate as a sign of narrative subjectivity and somatic and cultural resistance: "Baldness becomes me, in a literal sort of way, a hell of a lot better than a pink ribbon" (44).[7]

The photographs that Lord uses to introduce each section of her narrative appear without caption and range from self-portraiture to documentation of her medicalized status. The book's initial photographic representation of the writer's hair loss—a color close-up shot on the frontispiece of a glowing scalp, bald except for occasional brown follicles—jolts viewers who expect a conventional portrait featuring the subject's face and gaze.[8] Further indexical self-representation is withheld until the narrative's conclusion, when viewers confront a contact sheet that contains the original image and additional shots of the narrator's nearly bald scalp as her hair slowly diminishes. Intriguingly, the progression of hair loss and somatic revelation in this photographic sequence is nonlinear and visually unpredictable; the sixth frame, for example, arguably reveals more hair than does the fifth. Thus Lord subtly disrupts any facile desire on the part of viewers for a restitutive narrative from baldness to hair restoration.

The photographs that precede each chapter of *The Summer of Her Baldness* inscribe hospital treatment rooms and corridors as alienating

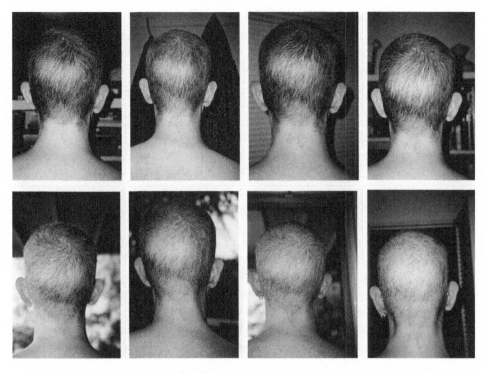

Untitled (detail). Courtesy of Catherine Lord.

technologized landscapes, occasionally mediated by a vase of flowers or a nurse's desk covered with computers, calendars, and framed family photographs. One photograph depicts the daunting entrance of a magnetic resonance imaging device; another presents an imposing rectangular chrome machine with multiple doors, elaborate tubes extending through various portals, and an indecipherable and almost comical sign handwritten in cursive and instructing absent medical personnel to "Remove Tubing Fri. PM (Or Thursday)" (9, 151). Other photographs capture similarly prescriptive signage, this time directed to patients: "If you are currently receiving chemotherapy, please double flush the toilet"; "NOTICE: IF YOU ARE PREGNANT, OR THINK YOU MAY BE PREGNANT, PLEASE INFORM THE TECHNOLOGIST PRIOR TO YOUR EXAMINATION" (95, 215). These signs remind viewers that biomedicine and the medical gaze are "disciplinary regimes" invested in surveillance and that patients are rarely accorded self-determination (Foucault, 1).

Lord represents the cancer patient's body as technologized terrain most dramatically in a black-and-white photographic juxtaposition of two mammography scans of her cancerous right breast. These slides contain impenetrable diagnostic scripting—"Lord Rt Med Breast 0/8 x 17 FFD = 145," and so forth—as well as the temporal marker 9-12-00 (205). The inability to decipher either the medical notations or the eerie gray shadings of the scans creates in many viewers an anxiety parallel to that of the patient. Furthermore, the scans' positioning in this photograph subtly parodies conventional media representations of women's sexualized breasts, since what would ordinarily be the nipple area is highlighted by a white diagonal line that lashes the black background and a narrow strip of what might pass as cleavage is evident between the two sides of the image. The need for surgical removal of the diseased portions of this technologically imaged breast is implicit in the photograph, which disrupts the breast's cultural sexualization by depicting it as the subject of medical intervention.

In addition to electronic commentaries and framing photographs, Lord's hybrid narrative incorporates email responses of friends in a wry dialectic that resembles a cross between a Greek chorus and a queer theory seminar. In response to Lord's email expressing her decision not to

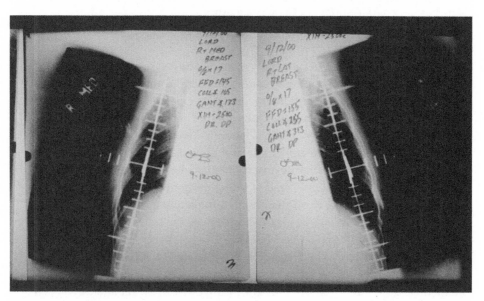

Scan. Courtesy of Catherine Lord.

"wig out" but to wear hats to conceal her hairlessness, a reader writes wittily, "Don't forget the new relationship is not only with your hats, but more importantly with your pate. HAVE A DATE WITH YOUR PATE!!" (38). In response to a highly theoretical email from Lord about cancer and medicalization, a friend identified as "WHYRAIN" replies, "JESUS Catherine, I always knew you were capable of the most Wittgensteinian ruminations, but baldness has apparently sent you into the philosophical ether" (42). As one friend teases Lord for overtheorizing her disease, another matches her excess. In response to a message entitled "Her Baldness Meets Beth and Gets High on Gender," Lord's listserv recipient "SEC" offers her or his own queer reading: "The gay men are all shaving their heads to mystify their balding/aging effects, so you were probably passing as a gay man, who was trying to pass as a young man. Just think, as you try to look more and more indecisive and 'girlish'—BUTCH BOTTOM!" (117, 123). With incisive wit and a rhetoric of gender bending, the members of Lord's email circle often one-up the primary narrator.

Like many postmillennial breast cancer narratives, *The Summer of Her Baldness* includes reflection on the U.S. cultural silencing of possible environmental factors in the current breast cancer epidemic.[9] In Lord's wry inventory of her breast cancer's likely causes she lists "chlorides, pollutants . . . chewing the fat of dead animals" along with her "melancholic disposition," her status as a lesbian who has never given birth, and her family history of two grandmothers who contracted this disease (26). Her implicit environmental critique focuses on carcinogenic treatment protocols: she reminds readers of the historic relationship of the chemotherapy agent Cytoxin to mustard gas in World War I, repeatedly likens her chemo cocktail to weed killer, and calls radiation a "carcinogenic beam" (48, 72, 117). What Lord's physicians refer to as her chemo "recipe" (the "perversely feminized metaphor oncologists prefer," she notes sardonically) is surely toxic: "Adriamycin and Cytoxan: they fit right in on the pesticide shelf" (48). Humor masks anxiety, of course. Even as Lord acknowledges the necessity of chemotherapy, she worries retrospectively about its harmful effects on Her Baldness, who "spent six months absorbing into her body substances invented by the military to make genocide more efficient" and thus can surely never be considered cured (171).

In her epilogue, a farewell letter to Her Baldness (now called H as a sign of her disappearing prominent status) written a year after the completion of her cancer treatment, Lord theorizes illness from a postmodern perspective, rejects once more the dichotomy of public versus private space, and interrogates the stigma and self-blame that accompany a breast cancer diagnosis. "I need to talk," writes Lord to her former amanuensis. "This is not to say that I miss you, because I can't decide whether I like you, but I am well aware that I owe you" (233). H invokes Lord's ambivalence not only because she evokes unwanted memories of traumatic cancer treatments but also because she exposes Lord's narcissistic response to illness: "Not only do you remind me of a time of fear and physical discomfort but you embarrass me. You spoke too loudly. . . . You pontificated. You patronized. You were bossy. You were prone to rage. You were maudlin. Sometimes you cried at the keyboard. You were greedy. You snarled" (235–36). Lord's linguistic excess serves as a tool for grappling with self-division, as she transfers to her imaginary doppelganger her fear, rage, and grief at her illness. Yet her whimsical representation of H suggests that this narrative persona understood early on what the cancer patient and writer analyzed only retrospectively—that illness as a social space infringes upon identity and recasts public-private boundaries.

> Illness is not something that happens to you but something you are—not someone's mother, for example, but the colon resection in room 235 that needs to be turned in the middle of the night. Illness is a transaction that involves other people, a lot of them. . . . Being ill can make you sicker than cancer. Illness is lonely, all the more so because it affords you no solitude. The so-called private pain of illness is in fact an observed, calibrated, measured, unremittingly public space. (236)

In this passage Lord theorizes illness as a vexed identity marker and medicalization as invasive technologized terrain. These insights were possible only through the invention of H as doppelganger, she concludes—a figure that served not only as her creator's alter ego but also as "a narrative device, a means to tell a story, a tool" (237).

Lord's breast cancer photo-narrative—feminist, queer, postmodern— openly identifies the performative strategies on which the writer-photographer relies. It also playfully interrogates gender, as seen in HB's musings on "whether the man of the house caught cancer or the femme between the sheets" (5). Multiple audiences bear witness to Lord's testimony through what philosopher Kelly Oliver terms "response-ability," an empathic form of listening that can hear an illness narrator into speech: intimate friends of Lord encourage her via email responses; her partner collaborates through dialogue included in the narrative; and readers of the published narrative who have never met its creator respond as part of the implicit contract Lord offers via her text's "reality effect" (Oliver, 15; Avrahami, 8). Ultimately *The Summer of Her Baldness* uses queer theory, strategic narcissism, and a postmodern rhetoric of indeterminacy to unmask the vulnerabilities of breast cancer patients and the self-reflexivity of postmillennial cancer narratives.

Marking Cancer's Contingent Embodiment:
Lynn Kohlman's Photo-narrative

After enduring a lumpectomy when her breast cancer was initially believed to be localized, a double mastectomy when her surgeon discovered cancer in her second breast, a delicate brain surgery for glioblastoma that resulted in staples being implanted and left visible in her scalp, and a recurrence of brain cancer two weeks later that necessitated massive radiation and years of grueling chemotherapy, Lynn Kohlman determined until her death in 2008 to "present herself as the beautiful public body of cancer," as one obituary put it (Horwell). Her written and visual assessment of the cancer experience in *Lynn Front to Back* presents it as both catastrophic and transformational: "Within a matter of seven months, I went from being healthy and whole to missing two breasts and having 37 titanium staples in my head. I needed to find my own inner source of strength and power. Maybe other people don't have to go through cataclysmic transformations for this kind of awakening to take place, but for me, that's what happened" (np). Such temporal markers as the phrase "within . . . seven months" appear often in this photo-narrative, unsurprisingly given the unusual speed with which Kohlman received diagnoses of two life-threatening cancers, but time constitutes just one of several textual markers. Other markers are spatial, as seen in the titular phrase "front to back." Still others are technological, for the experimental medical procedures that Kohlman endures produce a radically contingent body repeatedly marked up for surgery or radiation and visually marked (and remarked upon) thereafter.

Lynn Front to Back features commercial photographs and self-

portraits of the model turned photographer turned cancer patient; Kohlman's written account of the highlights of her personal and professional
life and her lived experience of cancer; photographs she took of famous
friends in the fashion world—Perry Ellis, Calvin Klein, Donna Karan—
alongside portraits of her husband, Mark Obenhaus, and their son Sam;
and testimonials by friends, family members, and associates that read ee-
rily like eulogies for a woman then still living. Kohlman's tone is resolute,
confident, and self-fashioning. "I never believed in my beauty as a model,
but here I am, 57 years old, with a double mastectomy, hair fried from
radiation, never feeling more beautiful! It's another shift, front to back"
(np). In her determination to redefine beauty in the face of catastrophic
illness and bodily trauma, she follows in the footsteps of Matuschka, the
U.S. model whose post-mastectomy photographic self-portrait *Beauty
Out of Damage* caused controversy when it appeared in 1994 on the cover
of the *New York Times Magazine* as a defiant step toward destigmatizing
breast cancer (Ferraro, 24–27).[10] Kohlman ups the representational ante
on Matuschka, however, by publishing an extensive photo-narrative, not
just isolated shocking photographs, and by baring repeatedly before the
camera's eye both her sutured chest and her surgically stapled skull.

One compelling representational strategy in *Lynn Front to Back* is
the text's initial juxtaposition, immediately following the title page and
Donna Karan's foreword, of two striking "then vs. now" photographic
portraits of Kohlman. Although neither photograph is titled or dated,
the representation of Kohlman's airbrushed face and nude torso by Barry
Lategan that appears on the left page clearly captures the youthful, sexualized model of the 1970s; her wide eyes gaze seductively at the camera,
her pixie haircut parted on the left is fetching, her breasts are full and
firm. The photograph of Kohlman on the right page, taken by Obenhaus
thirty years later, paints a radically different portrait of material embodiment, one that foregrounds the ravages of brain and breast cancer. Her
eyes, now melancholy, no longer face the camera's lens but gaze instead
into the distance; her thin forearms are bound by hospital tape, an IV
needle or portable catheter protruding from the bandage on the left.
For me, what Roland Barthes terms the *punctum* of a photograph—the
element that pricks, jolts, disturbs a viewer emotionally—is in this instance Kohlman's haircut, a kind of Mohawk necessitated by the semi-
circular metal staples that crown her half-shaved head at precisely the
line that the left part traced in the 1975 photograph. The postmillennial
photograph's *studium*—the meaning derived from its implied cultural

context—occurs via the temporal juxtaposition of hegemonically feminine breasts from 1975 and scarred, absent, gender-neutral ones from
2005, markers that signify surgical or technologized invasion (Barthes,
27–28). Kohlman's scarred chest jars viewers not just in its breastlessness
but also in its bold display of protruding ribs and its stark—is it possible to feel this?—*beauty*. Kohlman uses that noun frequently both in
her photo-narrative and in interviews following her surgeries to describe
the wounded body she embraces and displays, "determined not to hide
behind my scars": "I have finally realized, my breasts gone . . . I am beautiful" (np). Viewers may likewise relish the reconfigured iconography of
beauty that Kohlman's ravaged chest and sutured head assert, although
the autothanatographic implications of such ravages may create an ethically fraught response to this visual representation of a woman unlikely
to live much longer. As a model and a fashion ad designer, Karan notes,
Kohlman brought to her work an "androgynous street edge" (Karan, np).
The earlier embrace of a transgendered aesthetic accounts perhaps for
Kohlman's relative ease in redefining beauty through her wounded embodiment, as illustrated by the assessment she shares with Karan that
titanium staples made her look "elegant and edgy" and by the verve with
which Kohlman responds to the punk rocker who asks her admiringly
which famous hairdresser created her amazing haircut, "Dr. Holland at
Sloane-Kettering" (np).

As S. Lochlann Jain notes in her critical commentary on Kohlman's
cancer photographs, this subject's embodied and technologized markers
defy the facile pinkness of contemporary breast cancer culture: "These
scars display the trace of illness, the memorial of death" ("Cancer Butch,"
522). Kohlman's scars and staples remind viewers that many markers displayed on the bodies of cancer patients occur from invasive treatments
and technologies, not from the disease itself. Although Jain expresses
discomfort with the ways in which "Kohlman's images bring the mastectomy into an aesthetic of the beautiful death," she admires the photographer's decision to present her scars as "public, tough, and masculine";
their beauty, Jain contends, "lies not in the way they mark mortality but,
rather, in their hyperdesigned quality, in the way they draw attention to
the markings that technology leaves on the body" (522–24). While Jain's
analysis sheds valuable light on the breast cancer body as technologized
terrain, her claim that photographic images of Kohlman's scars contribute to "an aesthetic of the beautiful death" does not acknowledge sufficiently the subject's narrative testimony of her struggle to stay alive and

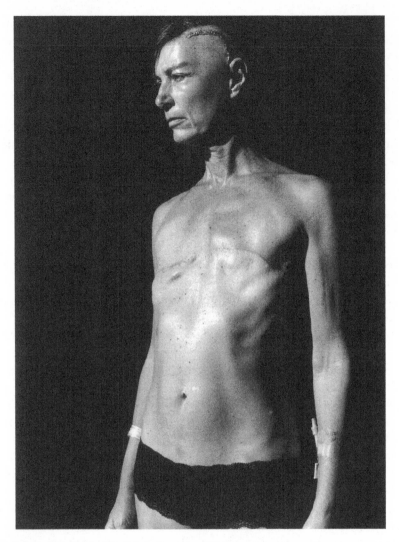

Mark Obenhaus, *Untitled*. Courtesy of the artist.

the trauma she experienced from the breast and brain cancers whose surgical treatment caused her scars.

Kohlman's technologized body provides the subject matter of another photograph by Obenhaus, *Radiation*, which depicts a figure that appears posthuman, scalp wrapped mysteriously in a net resembling protective fencing gear, marked up for brain radiotherapy and entering a massive treatment unit. This spectral photograph presents the cancer patient/subject, labeled Lynn Kohlman, prone, shrouded, and vulnerable. Its accompanying text, chosen by Kohlman, features an excerpt from Paolo Coelho's *Warrior of the Light* that emphasizes human suffering and resistance: "I carry with me the marks and the scars of battles— / they are the witnesses of what I suffered / and the rewards of what I conquered" (Kohlman, np). As noted below, such warrior discourse has a distinguished if vexed history in feminist cancer narratives; here Kohlman documents her resolve to endure invasive treatments in the hope of prolonging her life.

By her own admission Kohlman wished when young to become an artist rather than a model; she never felt comfortable as a glamorous photographic subject, yet she relished her location on the other side of the camera's lens. Her experience as a photographer gave her the courage to combat cancer, as she explains in the textual commentary that accompanies a photograph of the Rolling Stone's Keith Richards, his wild hair wrapped in a bandanna that covers a tan and wrinkled forehead, his smiling eyes gazing boldly at the camera.

> Photography. My timid nature dissipates, as I peer through my lens, making direct eye contact with my subject. . . . This intense sensation cuts to my core, and I feel joy, elation, and lightness; like flying. This experience is so explosive that, when faced with cancer, I knew that accessing this place within me would give me the strength to fight for my life. (np)

The fact that Kohlman sought courage as photographer rather than as photographic subject suggests the need for analytic focus not only on photographs taken of her by others but also on her cancer self-portraiture.

Self-Portrait with Expanders appears initially to represent merely the photographer turned cancer patient capturing her post-surgical image through the lens and a mirror. Her textual commentary, however, conveys Kohlman's indignation regarding the *studium* of this photograph, the prevalence of a male-dominant gaze and the fetishizing of large breasts in U.S. culture. Her flattened, post-mastectomy right breast appears to be growing in this photograph, while her left is slightly smaller but also puffy. Kohlman notes that although she agreed initially with her physician's recommended strategy of breast reconstruction, she encountered two problems: extreme pain during the process of reconstruction, and

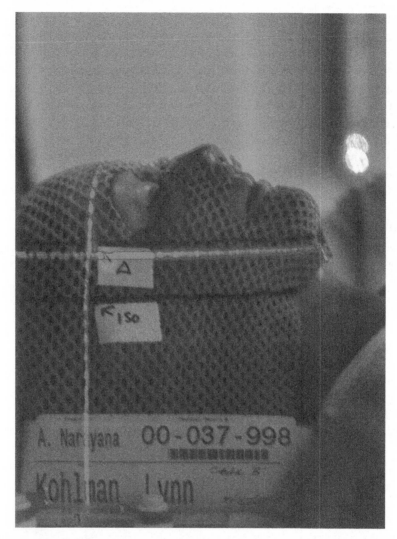

Mark Obenhaus, *Radiation.* Courtesy of the artist.

the surgeon's refusal to accept her decision to reduce her breasts rather than augment them. "Nobody had warned me how painful expanders could be," she explains; "it was like medieval torture every week, it was as if the screws were being turned tighter and tighter" (np). Furthermore, her breast surgeon was willing to implant only large breast expanders; when Kohlman objected that all along she had requested size 32B, she was informed that "the teardrop shape, smaller implants are not available in this country" (np). Outraged, she reports having challenged her surgeon to no avail, although she ultimately has the expanders removed and thereby resists hegemonic femininity and breast fetishization at the hands of her medical practitioner.

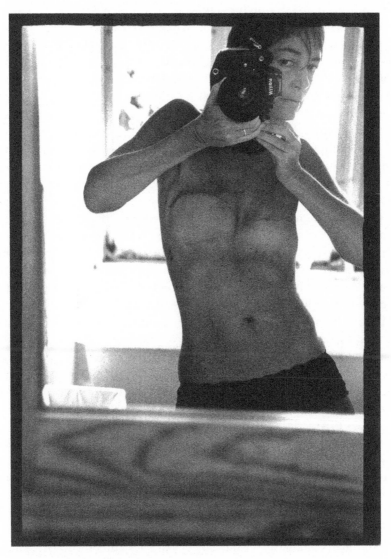

Lynn Kohlman, *Self-Portrait with Expanders*. Courtesy of Mark Obenhaus.

Kohlman acknowledges many other traumatic moments during her cancer struggles, most notably on a yoga retreat with Donna Karan and instructor Rodney Yee when she had "what I can only describe as an out-of-body experience. It was as if something was running up my spine, and I had this terrible taste in my mouth. Meanwhile, I was watching myself from someplace on the ceiling, looking down, feeling like I would never return to my body. I woke up screaming, shaking uncontrollably" (np). When the same sensations occurred the following day with Yee and Karan as witnesses, Yee proclaimed that Kohlman was experiencing kundalini rising. Kohlman demurred, aware that only yogis with many years of practice could reach such heights and that her seizures likely signified brain cancer, a diagnosis confirmed days later by her neurologist. To describe the resolve with which she confronts this new disease, Kohlman employs a rhetorical strategy used by previous cancer theorists from Susan Sontag in *Illness as Metaphor* to Audre Lorde in *The Cancer Journals*: a warrior discourse that the beleaguered patient adopts to gird her loins for battle against an encroaching enemy. Sontag, of course, famously critiques militant cancer metaphors; Lorde, in contrast, embraces warrior imagery, identifying it with the legendary Greek Amazons and with the one-breasted women warriors of Dahomey, her African homeland, from whom she drew courage to combat her illness (Sontag, 66–67; Lorde, 13–16). In her use of warrior imagery Kohlman departs from both the Western militaristic cancer discourse that Sontag challenges and the Amazonian imagery that Lorde adopts, choosing instead to imagine a samurai identity through which to combat her cancers: "I had been slammed to the ground and thrown down an abyss. Now I envisioned picking myself up and emerging a samurai warrior, sword in hand, ready for battle" (np). She explains this imagistic choice in pragmatic terms that often turn spiritual: "I already have western science covering me, and so, as in a battle, I needed to come in from the east. Whether I am on chemotherapy or not, I am on a concentrated regime of meditation and yoga to focus my breath and grab my soul; acupuncture and craniosacral therapy to normalize the flow of my energy as it courses through my body" (np). In choosing this holistic path she joins many contemporary cancer memoirists in detailing the meditative practices to which they turn in hopes of healing.

Kohlman's emphasis on the cancer patient's embodied agency foregrounds a perspective shared by Zillah Eisenstein in *Manmade Breast Cancers*.

My breast cancer body does not say enough about how other body demands have choreographed my life. Although breast cancer has often suffocated me . . . my body has had other selves. I am never simply my cancer because I have other bodies *and* I am something besides my body struggles. (42)

This manifesto reminds reader-viewers that Catherine Lord and Lynn Kohlman also have other bodies besides the ones represented in their photo-narratives, have had additional bodily demands in the course of their lives, are something besides their embodied struggles. Like Eisenstein, they invite audiences to invest them with full humanity.

Witnessing Breast Cancer Bodies and Testimonies

Feminist postmodern theory has long demonstrated that gendered bodies are never fixed but ever in process—multiple, contingent, and fluid. Since the body is both material and discursive, any feminist understanding of its corporeality must be mediated by its spoken contexts. As Judith Butler notes,

As an intentionally organized materiality, the body is always an embodying *of* possibilities both conditioned and circumscribed by historical convention. In other words, the body *is* a historical situation . . . a manner of doing, dramatizing, and *reproducing* a historical situation. ("Performative Acts and Gender Constitution," 272)

She thus contends that "there is no reference to a pure body which is not at the same time a further formation of that body" (272). How women's bodies have been constructed, objectified, politicized, and re-formed therefore becomes a central question for contemporary feminism and its visual and verbal representations of breast cancer. Indeed, the constructions of gender, technologized embodiment, and somatic resistance found in women's postmillennial breast cancer photo-narratives draw important links between "the everyday body as it is lived, and the regime of disciplinary and regulatory practices that shape its form and behavior" (Shildrick and Price, 8).

Because of the power and urgency that accrue to visual and verbal accounts of breast cancer, writers/photographers such as Lord and Kohlman infuse their photo-narratives with sociopolitical, ethical, and testimonial dimensions and engage readers and viewers as postmodern witnesses. Traditionally humans have borne witness when giving or hearing legal testimony, advancing spiritual claims, or revealing traumatic experiences, whether public traumas such as slavery, the Holocaust, and acts of genocide or private traumas such as rape, incest, or life-threatening illness. The concept of witness thus has juridical, religious, psychological, and medical histories as well as narrative status. As Oliver explains in *Witnessing: Beyond Recognition*, "the process of witnessing, which relies on address and response—always in tension with eyewitness testimony—complicates the notion of historical truth and moves us beyond any easy dichotomy between history and psychoanalysis" (2). Moreover, witnessing constitutes "the basis for all subjectivity," since becoming either a human or a narrative/discursive subject is a dialogic process that requires connectivity, a circulation of energies that constitutes a "fundamental ethical obligation" (715). As acts of visual or verbal subjectivity and witness that call in turn for reciprocal, or secondary, witnessing, contemporary breast cancer photo-narratives invite viewers and readers to embrace an imaginary identification with suffering and resistant others.

In Lord's *The Summer of Her Baldness* and in Kohlman's *Lynn Front to Back* this imaginary identification on the part of reader-viewers occurs through what philosopher Sara Ahmed terms the "emotionality of texts," which is "one way of describing how texts are 'moving,' or how they generate effects" (12). Textual emotionality occurs, she argues, through compelling narrative use of figures of speech, especially metaphor, which renders likeness, and metonymy, in which the part represents the whole. Lord's photo-narrative highlights Her Baldness not only as the narrator's grim double but also as a metaphor for the ravages of breast cancer diagnosis and treatment, whereas Kohlman's photo-narrative employs metonymy in its implicit titular equation of reading *Lynn Front to Back* and knowing its subject intimately. Emotional texts, Ahmed concludes, are both "sticky, or saturated with affect" and imaginatively grounding for readers: "What moves us, what makes us feel, is also that which holds us in place, or gives us a dwelling place" (11).

Avrahami notes in *The Invading Body* that reading or viewing an illness photo-narrative involves a collaborative process whereby cultural discourses intersect with a narrator's recollected representations of her corporeal experience to produce a contract between the autobiographical subject, discursive and provisional, and the reader-witness, who responds with some degree of "moral and rhetorical complicity" (20). *The Summer of Her Baldness* and *Lynn Front to Back* illustrate this ethical imperative well. Reading and viewing autobiographical/visual representations of breast cancer involve audiences, in Griselda Pollock's theoretical formulation, in "the process of moving from trauma to cultural memory" via artistic works that serve as talismans—as sites of somatic representation and remembrance that enable audiences to "lodge the pain of others in our memories" ("Dying, Seeing, Feeling," 234). As we encounter the postmillennial photo-narratives of Lord and Kohlman, reader-viewers thus serve as putative agents of witness and commemoration. In the chapters to come we shall consider further how theories and practices of testimony, spectatorship, and memory inform breast cancer narratives that focus on feminist activism, prophylactic mastectomy, transgressive humor, post-operative visual representation, autothanatography, and ethical remembrance.

2 | Audre Lorde's Successors
Breast Cancer Narratives as Feminist Theory

The compelling legacy of the self-described "Black lesbian feminist warrior poet" Audre Lorde (1934–92) has been the subject of significant critical commentary by theorists of breast cancer during the past decade. In *Beyond Slash, Burn, and Poison* Marcy Jane Knopf-Newman claims that both *The Cancer Journals* (1980), written shortly after Lorde's 1978 mastectomy, and *A Burst of Light* (1988), written after cancer had metastasized to her liver in the mid-1980s, catalyzed the work of feminist health activists: "Lorde's ideas motivated people to consider various modes of resistance to hegemonic ideas about women's bodies and women's health" (139). Activists have since paid tribute to Lorde in their organizational newsletters and websites, dedicated women's and gay health clinics in her name, and continued her project of "transforming silence into language and action" (Lorde, *Cancer Journals,* 18). Among the breast cancer crusaders who have acknowledged Lorde as a foremother are Dr. Susan Love, who in her *Breast Book* praises Lorde for having spoken out as a lesbian to control her treatment agenda; Barbara Brenner, former executive director of Breast Cancer Action, who quoted Lorde's writing for years in her organization's monthly publication as a way to inspire action; and Sandra Steingraber, poet and environmentalist, who urges contemporary feminists to join Lorde in "challeng[ing] the unquestioned and sanctioned discourse about what causes cancer" (Knopf-Newman, 139–40).

In a 2006 essay in *Signs* Diane Price Herndl evaluates Lorde's legacy as a breast cancer memoirist and characterizes her feminist analysis of the disease as unmatched by subsequent cancer narratives: "*The Cancer Journals* made an enormous difference not only in the visibility of breast cancer and in the possibilities of writing about it, but also in creating an imperative: not only should one write about one's experience of cancer, but doing so is a political act, and doing so correctly is an ethical act" (221). Although many contemporary memoirists have followed Lorde in making breast cancer visible, notes Herndl, most have not challenged prevailing medical or social codes, analyzed the role of environmental toxins on breast cancer, or explored the cultural politics of this disease (238). Herndl criticizes late twentieth-century breast cancer anthologies for their political quiescence, yet she rightly identifies two feminist theorists of cancer who did politicize the disease near the turn of the century: Eve Kosofsky Sedgwick, whose 1999 essay "White Glasses" theorizes connections between breast cancer and the AIDS pandemic, and Barbara Ehrenreich, whose 2001 essay "Welcome to Cancerland" indicts corporate promulgators of breast cancer culture for complicity in "global poisoning" (Herndl, "Our Breasts," 238–39, 242).[1] Although Sedgwick and Ehrenreich made valuable contributions to feminist cancer discourse, neither has published a cancer narrative comparable in scope to *The Cancer Journals*. It is therefore initially tempting to agree with Herndl that while some breast cancer narratives movingly depict private trauma, most of them fail to "look outward from this experience" (240).

In this chapter, however, I revise Herndl's contention by analyzing breast cancer narratives by three feminist mammographers whom I view as Audre Lorde's postmillennial successors: Zillah Eisenstein's *Manmade Breast Cancers* (2001), Evelyne Accad's *The Wounded Breast: Intimate Journeys through Cancer* (2001), and three essays by S. Lochlann Jain published between 2007 and 2010: "Cancer Butch," "Living in Prognosis: Toward an Elegiac Politics," and "Be Prepared." Like Lorde, these autobiographical theorists argue that breast cancer needs further feminist analysis and political scrutiny. All are academics—a politics professor, a novelist and poet who teaches languages, and a cultural anthropologist, respectively. Each writer contracted breast cancer in her thirties or forties; underwent mastectomy or lumpectomy, chemotherapy, radiation, and in two cases a second elective mastectomy; and determined to explore the disease from theoretical and experiential perspectives. All three writers acknowledge Lorde as a predecessor: Eisenstein praises her for having chosen "to be a militant one-breasted woman rather than practice what she felt was deceit" (32); Accad extols Lorde for having urged women to march on Washington to demand that Congress allocate more funding for breast cancer research; and Jain claims in "Cancer Butch" that *The Cancer Journals* "brought cancer out of two closets—the personal closet of disguise and the political closet of cancer production" (507).

The cancer narratives of Eisenstein, Accad, and Jain affirm yet extend Lorde's vision through six theoretical gestures.

1. They claim that breaking silence about breast cancer is still a vital feminist act but that new forms of silence exist to be broken.

2. They investigate probable links between breast cancer and environmental toxins, air and water pollution, food additives, and industrial waste.

3. They challenge the medical establishment, expose corporate control of the cancer industry, and interrogate the policies of mainstream organizations such as the National Cancer Institute (NCI) and the American Cancer Society (ACS).

4. They theorize the politics of appearance in breast cancer culture by questioning the emphasis on prosthesis, reconstruction, and hegemonic femininity.

5. They queer breast cancer by affirming lesbian or butch embodiment and resisting heterosexist assumptions that mainstream culture promulgates.

6. They assume antiracist and transnational perspectives in their analysis of breast cancer treatment and politics.

In the sections that follow I review Lorde's insights in *The Cancer Journals* and *A Burst of Light* and explore the ways in which her successors build upon her theories. I also consider ways in which they take issue with Lorde, thus disrupting any facile sense of an unmediated theoretical genealogy. In conclusion, I assess the cultural work that narratives by Eisenstein, Accad, and Jain accomplish and the breast cancer activist agendas that they offer for a postmillennial era.

Breaking New Silences

For Audre Lorde in 1980, speaking out about sexism, racism, and the politics and lived experience of breast cancer constituted a feminist ethical imperative. In her introduction to *The Cancer Journals* Lorde stakes her rhetorical and political claim.

Breast cancer and mastectomy are not unique experiences, but ones shared by thousands of american women. Each of these women has a particular voice to be raised in what must become a female outcry against all preventable cancers, as well as against the secret fears that allow those cancers to flourish. May these words serve as encouragement for other women to speak and to act out of our experiences with cancer and with other threats of death, for silence has never brought us anything of worth. (10)

Lorde draws here on the methodology of 1960s feminist consciousness-raising groups formed to help women hear each other into speech. Writing not only for herself but also for other women of all races, ages, and sexual orientations, she argues that truth-telling about "the travesty of prosthesis, the pain of amputation, the function of cancer in a profit economy" can help to liberate women from the confines of a racist, capitalist patriarchy (9). Linking silence to racism and heterosexism, Lorde challenges her readers to confront their own frightened visages: "What are the tyrannies you swallow day by day and attempt to make your own, until you will sicken and die of them, still in silence?" In stating unflinchingly her pedagogical purpose as "a black woman warrior poet doing my work, come to ask you, are you doing yours?" Lorde issues an impassioned call for women to question the troubling politics of breast cancer (21).

More than twenty years later, in *Manmade Breast Cancers*, Zillah Eisenstein states her narrative's purpose with similar explicitness but expanded reach: "Breast cancer is a political site from which I uncover the silences used to construct women's bodies. I share pain and suffering not simply to authenticate this way of knowing, but to push elsewhere" (ix). The elsewhere toward which she gestures is postmillennial global terrain, her chief metaphor that of traveling: "I begin with the breast and end with the globe *and* I start with the globe and end with the breast"—a paradox clarified by her claim that "my travels build a theorized journey from my body to a politics of bodies for a healthful globe" (x). Like Lorde, Eisenstein asserts transnational feminist consciousness as the lens through which she will investigate breast cancer; like Lorde, she embraces the ethical as well as the personal and/as the political, establishing for her narrative such goals as "personalizing the body politic" and "writing a female materiality" (4, 40). Eisenstein moves beyond Lorde, however, in focusing on the breast's wider environment, for a holistic approach to breast health demands "a rethinking of the politics of the body and the body of politics" (79). As a member of an Ashkenazi Jewish family deeply wounded by genetically influenced cancers—one sister died of breast cancer, another sister and an aunt died of ovarian cancer, and she and her mother have had breast cancer—Eisenstein nonetheless rejects simple or single causality, for in her view, genetic-centered narratives depoliticize breast cancer.[2] Like Lorde, she asserts that although there is no single breast cancer identity, most women who confront the disease grapple with issues of silence, invisibility, and fear. As a feminist theorizing cancer Eisenstein speaks for these women as well as for herself and her family: "I am humbled by the pain and grief and terror breast disease creates. I use this pain to push beyond the dominant narratives of nonseeing and silence" (x).

For Evelyne Accad in *The Wounded Breast,* too, narrating cancer in the twenty-first century's global contexts assumes both ethical and personal imperatives. Her narrative purpose is to reveal "the mutilations and deaths suffered the world over as a result of cancer" and to "help me overcome my anxiety and allay my fears," for writing ethically about cancer is both consciousness-raising and emotionally restorative (vii, 528). Moreover, in the poems, journal entries, and theories that she includes in this memoir, Accad connects the silence that surrounds an environmentally triggered breast cancer epidemic with other late twentieth-century massacres, one of which, the Israeli war against Lebanon, she and her family have experienced firsthand. She expresses concerns about the paucity and brutality of treatment options for women with breast cancer worldwide and asserts angrily after her mastectomy and radiation, "Before, I was proud of my body, but now I'm seeing it being mutilated, stitched up and mended" (221). Yet the drive to make meaning of her cancer remains paramount: "*What can I learn through this ordeal? What can it teach me?*" (14). Accad's queries recall Lorde's resolution in *The Cancer Journals* that "for other women of all ages, colors, and sexual identities who recognize that imposed silence about any area of our lives is a tool for separation and powerlessness, and for myself, I have tried to voice some of my feelings and thoughts" about the politics of cancer (9). Both writers thus acknowledge the therapeutic and pedagogical dimensions of narrating breast cancer.

Breaking new silences is also a goal of S. Lochlann Jain, who in "Cancer Butch" examines the effects of "butch phobia" on her own breast cancer experience and on mainstream cancer culture. She argues cogently that "there is simply no subject position available for cancer butch" in mainstream U.S. culture (521). Given this absence, a queer analysis is necessary to "provide a radical intervention into the ways in which gender is constituted and inhabited in relation to industrial capitalism and the distribution of one of its modes of suffering" (506). Extending Lorde's anticapitalist critique of 1980, Jain works to "untangle the motives of the breast cancer–corporate care nexus" from a postmillennial perspective (503). Her point of departure, a wry look at BMW's 2006 "Drive for the Cure" campaign, offers a rich vantage point for critiquing the corporate politics of the cancer complex. In addition, Jain join other contemporary theorists in challenging breast cancer culture's sentimental politics, pink iconography, and survivor discourses.

Connecting Breast Cancer to Environmental Carcinogens

Writing *The Cancer Journals* during the early stages of both the U.S. environmental movement and the women's health movement, Lorde seems prescient in having recognized that "cancer is becoming the physical scourge of our time" and that its likely causes are environmental: "My scars are an honorable reminder that I may be a casualty in the cosmic war against radiation, animal fat, air pollution, McDonald's hamburgers and Red Dye #2, but the fight is still going on, and I am still a part of it" (60). Anticipating the views of twenty-first-century holistic health advocates who recommend a vegan or macrobiotic diet as an antidote to cancer, she worries about the harmful effects on breast tissue of hormonally enhanced meats and chastises the ACS for its failure to make this problem visible: "Why hasn't the American Cancer Society publicized the connections between animal fat and breast cancer for our daughters the way it has publicized the connection between cigarette smoke and lung cancer? These links between animal fat, hormone production and breast cancer are not secret" (58). In support of this claim Lorde cites a 1978 study reported in the *British Journal of Cancer* and famously wonders "what would happen if an army of one-breasted women descended upon Congress" to complain about hormones added to beef, an act of mobilization that she unfortunately never enacted (*Cancer Journals*, 16). Yet throughout *The Cancer Journals* she laments "our environmental madness" and probes the carcinogenic aspects of "our malignant society," from cigarette smoke to car exhaust, from airborne chemicals to contaminated water (75).

Lorde extends her environmental critique in *A Burst of Light*, which chronicles her experience of traveling to Germany and Switzerland in the mid-1980s to seek holistic treatment for the cancer that had metastasized to her liver. In this book she reports on her dialogue with Swiss and German feminists about European studies linking breast cancer to chemical exposure: "Chemical plants between Zurich and Basel have been implicated in a definite rise in breast cancer in this region" (60). What frustrates her is the lack of power ordinary citizens have to control their own environments, much less to mandate corporate and governmental changes in environmental policy: "I'm not being paranoid when I say my cancer is as political as if some CIA agent brushed past me in the A train on March 15, 1965 and air-injected me with a long-fused cancer virus. Or even if it is only that I stood in their wind to do my work and the billows flayed me. What possible choices do most of us have in the air we breathe and the water we drink?" (120). Environmental irresponsibility is a form of terrorism, a claim that some readers might dismiss as extreme but for which Lorde makes no apology.

For Eisenstein, an emphasis on environmental factors in considering the worldwide rise in cancer incidences can challenge the genetic master narratives to which she has been subjected as a member of a cancer-prone family. As she clarifies in *Manmade Breast Cancers,* it is vital to "think of environments as plural and as entering the body" in ways that can lead to its contamination (ix). She uses the plural because environments are "rhizomed knots that often cannot be unraveled into singular sites" (84). Her particular concern in this regard is the potential hazard of tamoxifen and contaminated breast milk. With regard to tamoxifen, an antiestrogen medication widely prescribed to U.S. women with breast cancer and increasingly prescribed to high-risk women as a means of preventing the disease, Eisenstein points out that in 1996 the World Health Organization (WHO) identified it as a known human carcinogen, that its primary developer was the London-based Imperial Chemical Industries (later Zeneca, then Astra-Zeneca), which also developed and marketed carcinogens, and that the National Women's Health Network has questioned tamoxifen and its drug trials on three grounds: that it is difficult to determine which women are high risk, that small but significant numbers of cancer-free women have died while taking tamoxifen, and that the medication can increase the risk of ovarian cancer and blood clots.[3] With regard to breast milk, Eisenstein cites Steingraber's claim that it is the most contaminated human food due to the large amounts of dioxin found there, poisons that enter the body through air and water and then permeate the breast tissue and milk ducts.[4] Women's bodies are "the first environment," she concludes, and it is morally reprehensible that nursing infants at the age of six months have already internalized the amount of dioxin that scientists deem safe over a lifetime (148).

Eisenstein further analyzes the ways in which environments are socially constructed and the impact of carcinogenic occupations on the rise in breast cancer. "My notion of environments includes the knotted layerings that are unnatural, that are manmade, that construct the disregard for clean air, or fresh water, or healthy bodies," she explains. "Environments and diseases alike are socially constructed, although they also always contain remnants of what I hesitantly call their biogenetic potential" (84). Again quoting Steingraber, Eisenstein insists that "a cancer cell is made, not born" (155). One result is the creation of "cancer alleys" in towns such as Convent, Louisiana, the location of more than 140 petro-chemical and industrial factories and the home of many economically challenged residents, primarily African Americans or Latinos, who are subjected to high levels of toxicity and subsequently to high incidences of cancer and high rates of mortality (95–96).[5] Certain occupations have also long been identified as carcinogenic: the chromium industry, for example; most types of mining but especially uranium. Eisenstein cites the pioneering environmental research of Wilhelm Heuper in the 1950s and 1960s as well as the conclusion of Joseph Califano, U.S. Secretary of Health in the late 1970s, that "20–40 percent of all cancers could be caused by exposure to six industrial pollutants found in the workplace" (103).[6] Why have such arguments been marginalized in the early twenty-first century? she wonders, echoing a question Lorde asked decades earlier.

In *The Wounded Breast* Accad incorporates quotations from researchers who posit a correlation between the global rise in cancer incidence and environmental poisoning, most notably Steingraber but also French researchers Gilles-Eric Seralini and Lucien Israël. In her prologue Accad cites Steingraber's claim, supported by the World Health Organization, that 80 percent of cancers can be attributed to environmental influences. Early in her narrative Accad acknowledges, "I am but one of many people who have had to foot the bill for all the pollutants and chemicals ejected into the environment, which affect us through the air we breathe, the water we drink. . . . Our body can stand only so much of this sabotage" (13). The word *sabotage* recalls Lorde's fantasy of a CIA-transmitted cancer virus, and Accad uses similarly inflammatory diction throughout her narrative. As an immigrant to the United States she wonders whether she would have contracted cancer had she remained in Lebanon, given statistics revealing that once women from areas with low incidences of breast cancer live in the United States for several years their rates of contraction match those of U.S. women. "I'm paying the price of living in this civilization," she ruefully concludes (128).

Like Eisenstein, Accad is concerned with the impact of estrogen-producing toxins on breast tissue. She cites U.S. epidemiologist Devra Davis, who claims that women's greatest cancer risk comes from lifetime exposure to estrogen, whether from birth control devices or hormonally enhanced foods or ionizing radiation (316–17).[7] Indeed, when a friend suggests that "women's breasts are the receptors of the world's miseries," Accad concurs (261). As she consults with oncologists in the United States, France, Tunisia, and Lebanon, she gradually determines that her own cancer was likely triggered by the aggressive estrogen replacement therapy (ERT) that her gynecologist had prescribed to prevent osteoporosis, even though she was both premenopausal and asymptomatic (37–38, 67, 71, 259–60, 290).[8] In addition, she identifies the depletion of the ozone layer, the multiplication of pathogenic microbes worldwide, record levels of pesticides and industrial chemicals in drinking water, and high rates of urban pollution as explanations for the fact that while cancer has always existed, "it's manifesting differently and more aggressively, reaching epidemic proportions, and hitting younger and younger people" (164). By interweaving environmental scrutiny into her illness narrative Accad challenges the Middle Eastern belief system of her childhood, which posited that merely speaking the word *cancer* would bring on the disease (29). Probing the environmental causes of cancer allows Accad to de-stigmatize her disease.

In "Cancer Butch" Jain likewise insists on enhanced environmental scrutiny to assess breast cancer's causes and methods of prevention, and she indicts breast cancer fundraising strategies that protect carcinogen-producing industries. Using BMW as a case study, she notes that although this automobile manufacturer raised $9 million for breast cancer research through its 2006 Pink Ribbon "Ultimate Drive" campaign, the company's self-congratulatory publicity contained "no mention of the several known carcinogens that the car and gas companies have lobbied hard to allow in gas and car manufacture" (504).[9] Jain argues that "taking cancer seriously as an ethnographic object" will demystify corporate obfuscation of carcinogenic modes of production and demonstrate "the impossibly brutal underside of U.S. productive regimes."

Although corporations may like nothing more than to get rid of the ever-present threats that human cancers pose to production and consumption regimes (a dead smoker cannot buy cigarettes), at the same time the long incubation period [of cancer] and multiple possible causes provide a means by which causal relationships can be questioned. (506)

By questioning causal relationships between cancer and the carcinogens they produce, corporations can claim to have clean hands as they underwrite market-driven breast cancer philanthropy. As an antidote to such claims, Jain advocates for U.S. activist exposure of "the public violence of a culture in which fewer than ten per cent of its 85,000 chemicals are tested for carcinogeneity" (516–17). One way to combat this form of cultural violence is to view breast cancer as a communal rather than an individual disease—an approach that Lorde advocated and organizations such as Breast Cancer Action have long endorsed.

The activist memoirs of Lorde and her successors are therefore linked by an emphasis on environmental carcinogens, a connection established in the 1960s by Rachel Carson in *Silent Spring* but largely downplayed by the medical establishment even today. Such denial infuriates Eisenstein, Accad, and Jain, who view our carcinogenic environment as contributing to the rise of breast cancer worldwide.[10] Lorde puts it bluntly in *The Cancer Journals*: "Cancer is not just another degenerative and unavoidable disease of the ageing process. It has distinct and identifiable causes, and these are mainly exposures to chemical or physical agents in the environment" (73). It is not surprising that in her 2009 study *No Family History: The Environmental Links to Breast Cancer* Sabrina McCormick praises Lorde, along with Steingraber and Davis, as "sentinels to the new fight over breast cancer," women who have led others to "devote attention to the environmental *causes* of the disease in order to generate a new understanding of how to respond to the epidemic" (6). Clearly Eisenstein, Accad, and Jain likewise serve as sentinels whose writing is reshaping these debates.

Challenging Medical Hegemony

In *The Cancer Journals* Lorde chronicles her decision to take charge of her breast cancer treatment and recovery rather than accepting wholesale the advice of physicians. She explains why she insisted upon a two-step diagnostic process—biopsy first, mastectomy three days later—that was not standard procedure at the time and why she refused chemotherapy and radiation, which she considered carcinogenic. She lambastes the ACS and the NCI for suppressing research into the causes and prevention of breast cancer, and she coins the term *Cancer Inc.* to refer to the capitalistic medical system whose representatives pressure post-mastectomy women to wear prostheses, undergo breast reconstruction, endure grueling regimens of chemotherapy and radiation, yet blithely envision their post-operative selves as cured. In particular, Lorde accuses the ACS of colluding with the medical establishment to protect its economic interests by withholding information about holistic approaches to cancer. As the most powerful U.S. cancer organization the ACS should offer multiple perspectives on treatment, not merely that of conservative Western medicine, yet Lorde contends that the ACS fails to inform constituents about progressive alternatives.

> European medicine reports hopeful experiments with immuno-therapy, diet, and treatment with hormones and enzymes such as trypsin. Silencing and political repression by establishment medical journals keep much vital information about breast cancer underground and away from the women whose lives it most affects. . . . The ACS and its governmental partner, the National Cancer Institute, have been notoriously indifferent, if not hostile, to the idea of general environmental causes of cancer and the need for regulation and prevention. (72)

Ties to toxic corporations and the pharmaceutical industry, the concern of ACS board members and NCI employees to promote their own economic agendas, and a resistance to publicizing cancer information recommended by women's health groups are major factors in the failure of these agencies to serve constituents responsibly.

Lorde challenges insensitive medical personnel in *The Cancer Journals* as well as the medical hierarchy, most notably an oncology nurse who chides her for not wearing her prosthesis to a post-surgical consultation because a visibly one-breasted woman is "bad for the morale of the office" (59). Although she consented to a mastectomy, Lorde remained concerned that surgical interventions could activate otherwise dormant cancer cells; for this reason she refused exploratory surgery when doctors diagnosed a probable liver metastasis in 1984 and turned instead to holistic treatments such as injections of Iscator, a mistletoe-based biological believed to boost the immune system. "Every woman has a militant responsibility to involve herself actively with her own health," Lorde concludes. "We owe ourselves the protection of all the information we can acquire about the treatment of cancer and its causes, as well as about the recent findings concerning immunology, nutrition, environment, and stress" (*Cancer Journals*, 73).

In *Manmade Breast Cancers* Eisenstein updates Lorde's argument by critiquing a "transnational medicalized corporate structure" whose ideology prevents many physicians and researchers from envisioning "a science free to explore a holistic, interactive, and preventive modeling" of breast cancer (69). The argument that Eisenstein develops consists of ten areas that the medical establishment often fails to consider, including awareness that breast cancer is both an individual and a socially constructed disease, that mythologies of the breast and its cultural fetishizing negatively affect medical approaches to its diseases, that racism occurs in breast cancer treatment because the fetishized breast is "imaged as white," that breast cancer is underreported globally because economically vulnerable women have no access to health care, that breast cancer can confound oncologists because it "reflects and also constructs the medicalized gender visors of the historical moment," and that dominant estrogen narratives are misleading because "cancer cells, fed by estrogen, are viewed as self-determining rather than as a complex multifarious process of long-term mutations that interact with the body and its environments" (67–68).

Eisenstein rarely challenges the actions of particular doctors or nurses; rather, she identifies systemic problems fueled by a "petro/chemical-pharmaceutical/cosmetic complex" and a "postindustrial-medical complex"—powerful entities that affect the public's understanding of breast health through discourses developed to serve their own profit agendas (86). Seventeen percent of the U.S. economy is connected to medical services and/or the pharmaceutical industry, she notes; huge profits accrue to those who approach breast cancer as a disease that is genetically or estrogen-driven, and best prevented by estrogen-inhibiting drugs like tamoxifen—already a $320 million industry when she was writing in the late 1990s, nearly twice that today—rather than as an environmentally driven disease best prevented by eliminating workplace toxins, trace levels of DDT in soil, agricultural pesticides, hormones fed to cows and chickens, and plastics that mimic estrogen and disrupt normal hormone production (88–89). As Lorde did before her, Eisenstein exposes the corporate ties of key government agencies and cancer watchdogs, most notably the Federal Drug Administration (FDA), which "interlock[s] with pharmaceutical/drug companies to determine research initiatives and medical trials," and the ACS, whose board is made up of corporate donors (102). "Breast cancer is big business," Eisenstein concludes.

> Many of the same corporations that contaminate our bodily environments sell the drugs that are supposed to prevent malignancy. Zeneca manufactures pesticides at the one end and markets tamoxifen at the other. The postindustrial-medical/beauty complex researches and markets breast cancer at the same time. This just might be a deadly combination: moneymaking and women's health. (124–25)

In *The Wounded Breast* Accad castigates the medical establishment as well, concentrating particularly on physicians who fail to acknowledge their mistakes or who recommend invasive treatments that they know have little chance of success. "*What power doctors have over us,*" she laments (210). In the course of her treatment for a malignant breast tumor of three centimeters, the writer explains, she receives no apology from the gynecologist who prescribed the aggressive estrogen replacement therapy that might have triggered her cancer. Accad endures grueling months of chemotherapy recommended by an oncologist who later admits having known that it was unlikely to shrink the tumor, and she encounters another oncologist who blurts out that he "hasn't seen such a large tumor in four years" yet tells her not to worry (193). Although Accad praises one communicative surgeon, who performs her mastectomy and clearly explains her lobular carcinoma, she ultimately confides a loss of faith in modern medicine.

In a chapter entitled "Bureaucratic Doctors" Accad reports on a public lecture she attended in 1999 by an oncologist who recounted impassively the U.S. statistics on breast cancer—182,000 new cases would be diagnosed each year, 49,000 of which would be fatal—yet asserted that although U.S. women were high risk, few would want to live anywhere else, given the quality of life here. "*What quality of life, if breast and other kinds of cancer are on the rise?"* Accad wonders; *"What quality of life, if women have to undergo treatment that I consider to be 'twentieth-century torture'?"* (223). She notes that while the U.S. public typically (and justifiably) expresses outrage at torture conducted in their name during wartime, they fail to protest torturous medical interventions that "the 'developed world' inflicts on *itself*" (224). Bureaucratic oversight and physician indifference cause Accad to receive incomplete information about the risks her medical treatments carry; her radiologist, for instance, does not warn her about possible rib damage during radiation until she complains about brittleness in her chest bones, nor is she told until treatment is over that chemotherapy can trigger menopause.[11] During a costly consultation with oncologists at the Institut Gustave Roussy research center in Paris, Accad receives contradictory information: from one physician a disturbing diagnosis of the need for further chemo because her breast cancer is inflammatory rather than lobular, from another the claim that because her cancer is lobular and contained, further chemo would be ill advised. Since the two specialists never discuss their disagreement, Accad is left confused and disheartened. Like Lorde, she finally seeks holistic treatments, from Chinese herbs to mistletoe cream to relaxation therapy, and distances herself from the mainstream medical enterprise, which envisions women's ill bodies as "space into which the profit-making machine casts off its waste, as it casts off its waste into the rest of Nature" (500).

In "Cancer Butch" Jain likewise challenges the biomedical complex for its excessive attention to profitability and its long-term military links, as revealed through the history of the post–World War II development of radiation therapy, a treatment protocol that allowed the military to assess the effects of sustained radiation exposure on humans. She links the U.S. medical establishment to a "breast cancer–corporate care nexus" whose marketers urge consumers to buy pink kitchen products, breast cancer awareness postage stamps, and cosmetics designed to "offer the same redoublings of femininity that fissure through the entire biomedical complex of cancer treatments" (503–4). In addition, Jain finds it troubling that U.S. hospitals are structured as "a for-profit business, like selling raffle tickets or cheap candy" (511). As a Canadian living in the United States she endorses a government-run health care system that would provide equal access to care for all breast cancer patients. Toward the end of "Cancer Butch" Jain posits a question for postmillennial activists to probe: "How are we to understand this juncture of corporate care in liberal economies of gendered bodies in the context of a virtual explosion of the profitability of medicine?" (528). She goes on to indict the medical establishment for its greed and for its corporate and military ties.

Lorde, Eisenstein, Accad, and Jain thus share a narrative commitment to expose a systemically flawed medical establishment—an establishment that Lorde critiques as sexist, racist, and heterosexist; that Eisenstein considers governed by "carcinogenic capitalism"; that Accad accuses of "medicalized massacre"; and that Jain challenges for its connection to "the massive infrastructures of the military industrial complex" (Lorde, *Cancer Journals*, 72–73; Eisenstein, 100; Accad, 29; Jain, "Cancer Butch," 524).

Interrogating the Politics of Prosthesis and Reconstruction

The narrative moment that Lorde uses in *The Cancer Journals* to launch her critique of prosthesis is a post-mastectomy hospital visit she received from a volunteer with the ACS's Reach for Recovery program, a potentially valuable support service undermined by its emphasis on conventional femininity and cosmetic concealment. This woman's message— "You are just as good as you were before because you can look exactly the same. Lambswool now, then a good prosthesis as soon as possible, and nobody'll ever know the difference"—offends Lorde for its focus on appearance rather than survival, its assumption that only two-breasted women can look attractive, its corollary assumption that all post-mastectomy women are heterosexual, and its expectation that to look and feel the same after breast cancer would be positive for women rather self-denying (42). Lorde declares emphatically, "I refuse to hide my body simply because it might make a woman-phobic world more comfortable" (60). She further argues that by wearing prostheses women participate in their own silencing, invisibility, and infantilization: "By accepting the mask of prosthesis, one-breasted women proclaim ourselves as insufficients dependent upon pretense. We reinforce our own isolation and invisibility from each other, as well as the false complacency of a society which would rather not face the results of its own insanities" (61).[12]

Lorde is equally resolute on the then-new topic of breast reconstruction, which she labels an "atrocity . . . now being pushed by the plastic surgery industry as the newest 'advance'" (68). She emphasizes reconstruction's potential dangers, high cost, and cosmetic rather than curative nature, and she critiques physicians who urge women to undergo reconstructive surgery as a way to become whole. While she does not condemn individuals who choose prosthesis and/or reconstruction, she questions how free such a choice is since the U.S. public is "surrounded by media images portraying women as essentially decorative machines of consumer function, constantly doing battle with rampant decay" (64). Lorde brands as misogynistic surgeons who recommend that women reconstruct both their healthy and their cancerous breast to attain symmetry, since cosmetic surgeries are always medically risky. Ultimately she rejects reconstruction and prosthesis on the grounds that they prevent emotional well-being: "Either I would love my body one-breasted now, or remain forever alien to myself" (44).

Writing in 2000, when breast reconstruction had become commonplace (estimates suggest that up to 60 percent of U.S. women who have mastectomies now undergo this procedure), Eisenstein explores the politics of prosthesis and reconstruction from a different vantage point than Lorde's, yet she too questions the cultural assumption that cosmetic enhancement is desirable.[13] Because her cancer had a likely genetic component, Eisenstein reports having chosen prophylactic surgery on her right breast months after a mastectomy removed her cancerous left breast; like Lorde, she refused reconstructive surgery. In her narrative Eisenstein criticizes her oncologist for pushing reconstruction: "I wondered why she was so much more focused on the cosmetics than on the recurrence of cancer for me" (27). Explaining her choice to "map my own cancer look" by exercising with weights to strengthen her chest muscles, Eisenstein revels in running defiantly topless but acknowledges wearing a breast prosthesis occasionally "as costume" (31–32). While she praises Lorde for her political stance, Eisenstein differs with her predecessor about the ethics of prosthesis and reconstruction.

> I wish I could talk to Audre Lorde about this now. . . . She asserted her one breastedness in order to make breast cancer visible. Lumpectomy has of course changed the issue of (in)visibility. . . .
>
> It is many years later and I am not sure there is one truth or form of militancy today. . . . I have reconstructed my own body while my body is never wholly mine to define. I have chosen my flesh over silicone or saline, but sometimes this is not enough. So I clearly do not want a breast cancer identity plastered onto me. (32–33)

Eisenstein's perspective reflects postmodern assumptions about embodiment: an acceptance of bodily hybridity, an awareness of multiple and contingent identities, and ambivalence toward a definition of feminism that would require women always to make visible their breast cancer status.[14]

Accad reports in *The Wounded Breast* that she usually wears a prosthetic device, although she expresses ambivalence about her choice. Late in her memoir she admits that while a part of her would prefer to reveal her one-breastedness to the world, she chooses the easier alternative, concealment; she does not analyze this decision, only complains about the cost and discomfort of prosthesis. Accad expresses mixed feelings about reconstruction as well. On the one hand, she resents the cultural pressures that urge women to reconstruct their breasts as an homage to conventional femininity: "I have strong feelings about the artificiality of reconstruction, and especially about the discourse that surrounds it" (526). On the other hand, "I still feel mutilated in my body . . . off balance; as embarrassed and uneasy as a person would be after he or she had lost a limb. This is why I occasionally pay a visit to a plastic surgeon. As yet, I haven't resolved the problem" (527). Like Eisenstein, Accad cites Lorde in her discussion of whether to remain one-breasted. Having found *The Cancer Journals* "painful to read because the author suffers so much," she nonetheless praises Lorde's political vision: "I enjoy engaging with her because she's politically aware of the disease" (150–51). Despite her acknowledged sense of disfigurement, Accad commissions a friend to photograph her post-operative body, and she displays on the cover of her memoir a gripping image of her bald head, puckered mastectomy scar, and remaining breast as she confronts the camera with a sober gaze. This friend also photographs Accad with a sister cancer patient, Severine Arlabosse, as the two smiling women reveal their scarred chests and the heads they shaved to prepare for hair loss from chemotherapy. Accad includes these images in her narrative as an antidote to cultural denial and environmental myopia. "Why are women so quiet about their suffering?" she wonders. "Being photographed is a way of dominating my anxieties and fears, for me to say 'Look at me; I'm here. This is what you did to me, how your poisoned civilization poisoned my breast—invaded my whole body with its mad cells'" (208–9).

As a queer theorist and a cancer butch Jain expresses ambivalence not toward prosthesis or reconstruction but toward breasts themselves, for as gendered bodily markers, breasts "forced me to live in a sort of social drag" ("Cancer Butch," 514). The arrival of breasts at puberty, she explains, initiated unwelcome social expectations of gender conformity; while she never wanted to "be a guy," neither did she wish to be socially constructed as feminine (514). Although Jain confides that after her cancer diagnosis she initially felt dismay when viewing photographs of women's post-mastectomy chests, once she recovered from surgery she began to consider prophylactic mastectomy on her remaining breast.

> For months after my first mastectomy but before the second, I repeatedly found myself in the mirror: apprising with clothes off, with clothes on. With a shirt on I wanted the second breast off, with the shirt off I wanted the breast on. (512)

Eventually she recognizes that a second mastectomy would offer "an opportunity to have my body approximate, albeit inexactly, my body image," and after undergoing elective surgery she admits that "having no breasts seems illicit, although neither pleasure nor shame covers the range" (514). While she takes pleasure in her newfound ability to hold her children close to her chest, she acknowledges struggling to feel comfortable in a public culture that stigmatizes butches *and* breastless women. At one point in "Cancer Butch" Jain recounts a spontaneous decision to remove her shirt during one yoga class and expose her scarred chest—a gesture that she deems "a bow to Audre Lorde" for her public challenges to prescribed gender norms: "Can women not show their chests in public because they are women, or because they have breasts?" (515). While Jain's disrobing does not answer this query, it does offer, in her view, "a tiny, hard resistance to the layering of social shame on the experiences of cancer" in a heterosexist public sphere (515). She removes her shirt because she wants her breast cancer body "witnessed as a material artifact that visibly bore what I have always understood to be the public violence of a culture" that refuses to test ninety percent of its pharmaceuticals and other chemical products for toxicity (516–17).

Although Jain pays tribute to Lorde as a pivotal breast cancer theorist, she finds it problematic that many contemporary feminists regard her positions on prosthesis, reconstruction, and activism as iconic, for both mainstream cancer culture and attitudes toward breast conservation and reconstruction have shifted in the decades since *The Cancer Journals* was published. Postmillennial feminists should acknowledge, Jain concludes in "Cancer Butch," that "HIV/AIDS activism, a revolution in thinking on gender brought about by queer theory, and the inklings of new approaches to a cancer aesthetic, have changed the stakes of the public and private in thinking through the shame, illness, and sexuality nexus" (507). She thus reshapes Lorde's vision of defiant breast cancer embodiment for the twenty-first century by queering it.

Queering Breast Cancer

In recounting the story of a Reach for Recovery hospital volunteer who brought Lorde a pale prosthesis to wear after mastectomy, she exposes the woman's heterosexism as well as her racial myopia. Losing a breast "doesn't really interfere with your love life," the volunteer informed a bemused Lorde, who confesses in *The Cancer Journals* that although she "didn't have the moxie or the desire or the courage maybe to say, 'I love women'" when the volunteer asked if she was married, she would surely never worry about heterosexual beauty norms (42–43). Lorde's concerns are how to survive and prevent a recurrence, not how to cope sexually, for "a lifetime of loving women had taught me that when women love each other, physical change does not alter that love. It did not occur to me that anyone who really loved me would love me any less because I had one breast instead of two" (56). She thus refutes heteronormativity by defining a lesbian post-mastectomy erotic.

Lorde further bemoans the lack of visible lesbian role models for breast cancer patients in 1980. She acknowledges wishing that she could "share in dyke-insight" about her mastectomy, and she questions the invisibility of lesbians of color in the leadership of breast cancer organizations: "I wonder if there are any black lesbian feminists in Reach for Recovery?" (42, 49). In foregrounding lesbian identity and sexuality as central to her cancer experience Lorde never fears that her lover will reject her, but she wonders in her journal how lovemaking will differ now that she is one-breasted: "I was thinking, 'What is it like to be making love to a woman and have only one breast brushing against her?' I thought, 'How will we fit so perfectly together ever again?'" (43). Yet even as she mourns the loss of her breast, she recognizes that its erotic power can still be tapped: "Right after surgery I had a sense that I would never be able to bear missing that great well of sexual pleasure that I connected with my right breast. That sense has completely passed away, as I have come to realize that that well of feeling was within me" (77). In *A Burst of Light* Lorde again writes as a lesbian feminist determined to approach cancer as one of many political struggles: "Battling racism and battling heterosexism and battling apartheid share the same urgency inside me as battling cancer" (116).

Challenging heterosexism is a prominent topic in Jain's breast cancer narratives as well, although her queer postmodern approach differs from Lorde's lesbian feminism. In "Cancer Butch" Jain queers breast cancer by focusing on the lack of a subject position for butches in contemporary cultural cancer discourses. "What are the idioms that a cancer butch gets to inhabit?" she wonders, given the heterosexism of mainstream breast cancer culture (516). By defining her theoretical project as "disentangling the alliance between breasts and gender," she invites readers to ponder "how their disengagements have been marked and framed through various modes representing beauty, shock, and shame" (507). Like Lorde, who complained in 1980 about her post-mastectomy hospital visit from an ACS representative hawking cosmetics, fashion, and hegemonic femininity, Jain challenges Estée Lauder's "Look Good, Feel Better" campaign, whose literature appears in U.S. hospital oncology wings, mammography clinics, and doctors' waiting rooms. Looking good still translates as being feminine and heterosexual, Jain contends; mainstream breast cancer culture continues to depict as its iconic survivors young women wearing glamour wigs, breast prostheses, and tight pink T-shirts. Just as Lorde once "bristled at the way in which her lambs' wool prosthesis was intended to make her appear whole again," Jain rejects the postmillennial version of reconstructed breasts and examines how and why "the absence of the breasts introduces a new set of interpretive problems for the odd mix of gender and illness, internal and external health and appearance, that cancer and its cultures presents" (516).

Having decided to begin what she calls "my own personal Anti–Look Good campaign, a campaign in which hair and eyebrows were overrated," Jain wittily claims breastlessness and baldness as butch-inflected insignia of wholeness. Yet she notes in "Cancer Butch" that despite such queer campaigns, mainstream culture continues to place transgendered cancer patients in untenable positions.

> The public coding of breast cancer provides a strange intergendered space such that the butch woman literally cannot be tough

in "battling" cancer, and still maintain a gender identity as a butch. Not wearing the wig, for example, results not only in being a bad cancer patient but also gets coded as aggression. So how can one maintain her investment in performing toughness, let alone recuperate butchness, in the sea of pink designed precisely to "heal" by restoring and recuperating a presumed "lost" femininity? (521)

This question leads Jain to theorize breast cancer's gender coding as discriminatory toward those who reject heterosexual norms. Thus, even as she decries the absence of any "subject position available for cancer butch," Jain carves out its terrain (521).

In *The Wounded Breast* Accad does not address lesbian invisibility or heterosexism to the extent that Lorde and Jain do. Although she describes attending lesbian-feminist events, mourning the breast cancer diagnoses of lesbian friends, and mentoring gay youth during a visit to Beirut, queer discourses do not figure prominently in her narrative. Eisenstein does explore the disease's queer politics in *Manmade Breast Cancers*, questioning the logic, for example, of established medical claims for lesbians' heightened cancer vulnerability.

> It is often said that lesbians are at higher risk for breast cancer because they do not bear children. Of course this assumes that lesbians have not had children, which is very often not the case. So is the assumption of lesbian high risk simply, an assumption, or is there evidence to the contrary? As well, if lesbians are found to have higher cancer rates, is it not possible that one's economic status is also in play here? Maybe some lesbians suffer the absence of male wages like poor women more generally. (120)

In this passage Eisenstein challenges the stereotype of lesbians as childless, introduces issues of lesbian identity and economic justice, and challenges researchers to do smarter research on sexuality and breast cancer. In addition, she echoes Jain in arguing that not all breast cancer patients view loss of breasts as negative: "One sees this deep imprint of breast culture maybe most clearly with people who reject the clarity of heterosexist categories of identity. For female to male transsexuals, mastectomy is experienced as freedom" (136). By acknowledging multiple gendered perspectives on post-mastectomy embodiment, Eisenstein joins Lorde and Jain in queering breast cancer.

Resisting Racism, Thinking Transnationally

In *The Cancer Journals* Lorde bears witness to racialized bodies under siege, whether from the Holocaust or lynch mobs, apartheid or cancer. In *A Burst of Light* she makes transnational links explicit: "The devastations of apartheid in South Africa and racial murder in Howard Beach feel as critical to me as cancer" (11). An antiracist stance is evident throughout *The Cancer Journals,* as Lorde challenges white feminists who fail to recognize that "the blood of black women sloshes from coast to coast" and laments the deaths of Black youth due to racist violence (11–12). She is further outraged by an article in which a physician claims that only unhappy people get cancer: "In this disastrous time, when little girls are still being stitched shut between their legs, when victims of cancer are urged to court more cancer in order to be attractive to men, when 12 year old Black boys are shot down in the street at random by uniformed men who are cleared of wrongdoing . . . what depraved monster could possibly be always happy?" (75). Only those who work for social justice can experience even momentary joy, and it provides no insulation from suffering.

Extending Lorde's analysis, Eisenstein in *Manmade Breast Cancers* critiques white patriarchy for enforcing gender and racial privilege and develops an "anti-racist . . . feminist episteme" for analyzing how racism makes invisible both violence against women of color and their cancers (141). She notes that U.S. cancer rates are highest in communities populated by poor people of color, who suffer disproportionately from heavy pesticide use in public housing, exposure to toxic waste dumps that wealthy communities have rejected, and soil contamination by agribusiness; environmental racism exists because of racial and class privilege that leads to zoning inequities, she argues. Eisenstein especially strives to understand why black women in the United States have a higher mortality rate from breast cancer even though white women experience higher incidences, and she rightly claims that "late-stage diagnosis and lack of medical access, an intimate part of the politics of racism, define the varied realities of breast cancer" (97). She cites the research of epidemiologist Nancy Krieger, which reveals that black women under forty experience particular risk of breast cancer, as do highly educated black women, and she proposes more extensive transnational research on breast cancer, race, and racism.

Accad, too, evinces a global feminist consciousness in *The Wounded Breast,* expressing solidarity with those who have suffered "mutilations and deaths . . . the world over as a result of cancer" (vii). She praises Middle Eastern women who have written about cancer, most notably the Lebanese poet Nadia Tueni, who died in 1983, shortly after publishing her collection of poetry *July of My Remembrance*. In her chapter "Breast Cancer in France: Why So Hushed Up?" Accad cites examples of cultural silencing and trivialization of the disease and probes its possible causes. Most controversially, she compares Holocaust victims and breast cancer patients, noting that women today are often blamed for contracting breast cancer due to stress or poor diet, just as Jews in Nazi Germany were blamed for the anti-Semitism that led to their extermination. While Accad acknowledges this comparison as inflammatory, especially because she writes as an Arab woman, she argues that both the Holocaust and the breast cancer epidemic serve as "paradigm[s] of modernity gone horribly awry" (31). In addition, she employs cancer as a metaphor for Israel's 1996 bombardment of her homeland—"this blight is like a cancer coming back into Lebanon, my dear country"—and argues that military bombing and chemotherapy share common ground.

> Both total warfare and some of these all-out, aggressive cancer therapies serve only to shift the problem from the source to the symptoms. Both situations are preventable, and both are an expression of failure to resolve imbalances while there's still time. Cancer and wars of mass destruction are the hallmarks of this century, and of a world that's bursting at the seams with contradictions and conflict that continues to spiral. (471)

Despite her apocalyptic rhetoric, Accad draws convincing parallels between her amputated breast and her wounded country.

Although Jain's essays do not emphasize the global dimensions of breast cancer, as a Canadian she sometimes compares her country's cancer culture to that of the United States. In "Cancer Butch," for instance, she lambastes the Breast Cancer Fund of Canada for its sexist use in breast self-examination advertisements of a predatory teenage-male cartoon figure called Cam who offers to examine girls' breasts free of charge: "Playing on a long-standing joke of adolescent boys, the primary violence of the ad is its collaboration—even in its purported goal of early detection—in the same logic that has belittled the disease. Is any other medical procedure sexualized in this way?" (525). However, she extols the Canadian government for presenting photographs of lungs blackened from cancer as part of its public antismoking campaign. By extending her analysis to Canada, Jain reminds readers that both hegemonic and radical advertising initiatives cross borders, just as the disease of breast cancer does.

Extending Lorde's Vision

What textual and cultural work do the breast cancer narratives of Eisenstein, Accad, and Jain perform? How do they extend Lorde's vision, and what models do their critiques of mainstream breast cancer culture offer postmillennial readers and activists?[15] Like Lorde, Eisenstein foregrounds transnational feminist perspectives by asserting the "materiality of the female body as a site for resistance against human degradation and global obscenities" and by contextualizing breast cancer activism worldwide.

> When women in Islamic countries defy interpretations of the sharia that they know to be unjust, when women in Cuba demand lesbian rights, when women in Nigeria lead the movements against environmental degradation, when women in Pakistan, and India, and South Africa demand better medical access for dealing with breast cancer, they are all speaking from their localized bodies and their cultural meanings that voice a shared experience across the globe. The pull and seductiveness of feminism derive from the truths of bodily experiences. (154)

In "taking the breast to the globe," Eisenstein envisions a geopolitical feminism that would challenge the oppression of women across borders and affirm women's ownership of their bodies as "transversal" (151–53). In addition, she reports the findings of women with whom she interacted at the 1999 Second World Conference on Breast Cancer regarding lack of access to first-rate treatment protocols, medications, and prostheses as well as the stigmatization they confront (161–66). Ultimately Eisenstein affirms that a valuable new "racialized gender politics emerges as family, nation, and globe are renegotiated" (151–55).

Accad shares the ethical imperatives of Lorde and Eisenstein with regard to radical cancer activism. Breast cancer incidences are rising and the disease increasingly affects a younger population.

> We must make the facts known to the world so that both today's and tomorrow's generations will know, and so that women who have been hit by the disease won't be forgotten, as so many of their silent sisters have been who've never opened their mouth because they're told to be quiet, or who are never given a chance to speak; or who have their mouth shut as a result of centuries of crushing, sewing up, veiling, masking and closing up. (16)

Speaking out about the inadequacies of breast cancer's current treatments constitutes for Accad a global feminist intervention and a way to commemorate women silenced by breast cancer and other bodily violations.

As an antidote to shame and self-blame, Jain encourages postmillennial cancer activists to adapt militant strategies used by cycling rights and HIV/AIDS organizations. In "Cancer Butch" she envisions an approach that would take its cues from anti-car activists' "ghost bike" initiatives in which protesters chain white bicycles to sites where cyclists have been killed, and she praises members of Act Up for their radical acts of resistance: "They rioted, they educated, they stormed the National Institutes of Health, they unleashed power and they were arrested and they made news" (527).[16] Jain expands this argument in "Be Prepared" by urging cancer organizations to protest legal carcinogens rather than proffer sentimental discourses of hope.

> What if instead of some broad and grammatically, if not affectively, meaningless aim as marching and riding "for hope," fundraisers attempted to ban any one of the thousands of known carcinogens in legal use? What if we walked, ran, swam, rode not for hope, but against PAH, MTBE, BPA or any other common carcinogen? Such an effort would require naming the problem rather than the symptom, and recognizing how we are all implicated. It would require that we invest in cancer culture not as a mode of sentimentality but as a basic fact of American life. (181)

Although activism remains critical, public confrontation with suffering and grief is also essential. In "Cancer Butch" Jain advocates an elegiac cancer politics that would "proliferate the possible identities of illness—including dying" (506).

Rather than a call to action, an elegiac politics recognizes the basic human costs of U.S.-style capitalism. The point is not simply to eradicate the shame that has for centuries accompanied the disease, but also to acknowledge the ugliness of the disease and of the suffering it causes. . . . I draw a space in which cancer can be brought out of the closet in a way that is not about comforting ourselves and each other, and that is not about righteous anger but, rather, is a space of mourning and a space that allows for the agency and material humanity of suffering and death. (506)

A cancer culture that privileges survivorship does injustice to the dead and dying, Jain contends, by feeding discourses of disavowal.

Eisenstein, Accad, and Jain are allied with Lorde in endorsing militant forms of cancer activism, even as they reconfigure her vision for a postmillennial era. Their narrative delineations of feminist, environmental, transnational, queer, and anticorporate perspectives represent major theoretical challenges to contemporary cancer culture. Such narratives remind readers that all autobiography, especially political memoir, involves a complex intersection of the writing subject's discursive position, embodied materiality, and sociohistorical location, and that breast cancer offers a productive critical site for both self-disclosure and cultural intervention.

3 | Narratives of Prophylactic Mastectomy
Mapping the Breast Cancer Gene

In *Manmade Breast Cancer* Zillah Eisenstein offers not only a feminist manifesto but also a genealogical narrative of her family's illness history: "I want to go deeply into my body's story, which is entwined with my mother's and sisters' bodies. . . . If there is such a thing as genetically inherited breast cancer, I most probably have it" (1–4). Her mother, Fannie Price Eisenstein, contracted breast cancer during the 1960s at age forty-five but, after a radical mastectomy, survived into her eighties. Eisenstein's older sister, Sarah, and her younger sister, Giah, were less fortunate; both were diagnosed in their mid-twenties, underwent mastectomies followed by chemotherapy, lived free of cancer for several years, then learned that the disease had returned. Sarah's breast cancer metastasized in her lungs and finally spread to her brain, while Giah contracted cancer in her second breast and had another mastectomy, only to be diagnosed several years later with stage-four ovarian cancer. Despite extensive medical treatment, both sisters died in their thirties. At her doctors' urging, Eisenstein had a prophylactic oophorectomy shortly after Giah was diagnosed; following her sisters' deaths she contracted stage-one breast cancer, underwent a mastectomy followed by chemotherapy, and ultimately had a preventive mastectomy on her remaining breast. "Giah's second breast cancer weighed heavily in this decision," Eisenstein explains. "My cancer was lobular, which often means it will occur bilaterally. I did not want to risk another round of chemo down the road" (30). As of 2000, Eisenstein had remained cancer free for twelve years and had elected not to be genetically tested, despite the fact that Giah had tested positive for the BRCA1 mutation. Although Eisenstein acknowledges genetics as a factor in her disease, she finds disturbing the reigning medical assumption that the cause of breast cancer in the 5–10 percent of women who are BRCA-positive is their genetic makeup. "Knowing Giah had the BRCA1 mutation makes everything seem more fixed than it is," she argues. "The gene is a predisposition but not for all women who carry it. I think you never know if it is the gene or the triggers to the gene that are the culprit" (37).

Eisenstein's is one of a growing number of autobiographical narratives that chronicle women's experiences with inherited breast cancer and their decisions to undergo prophylactic mastectomies; in some cases the illness saga also includes ovarian cancer and preventive oophorectomies.[1] Many memoirists reveal less skepticism than Eisenstein, however, regarding the necessity of genetic testing and the role that genes play in the cancers that plague their family members.[2] Indeed, they view genetic predisposition as both the reason for these familial cancers and a threat to themselves, and they consider prophylactic surgery a reasonable or an essential form of protection, even if they have not been diagnosed with breast cancer.[3] What has happened in recent decades, scientifically, medically, and culturally, to lead women with breast cancer in their families to seek genetic testing, to have their breasts removed upon testing positive for a genetic mutation, and, in certain cases, to document their family histories and their own surgical experiences in multigenerational memoirs?

Mammographies that foreground prophylactic mastectomies are largely a postmillennial phenomenon, since the research that made genetic diagnoses possible is only two decades old. In 1990 geneticist Mary-Claire King discovered a gene connected to hereditary breast cancer, located on the long arm (q) of chromosome 17, thus confirming oncologists' long-held beliefs that certain cancers clustered in families. By 1994 Mark Skolnick and his colleagues at Myriad Genetics, a biotechnology company in Utah, had determined the precise DNA sequence of BRCA1, the name given to the gene that King had identified; a second gene, BRCA2, was located in 1995.[4] Mutations in these tumor suppressor genes sometimes produce defective proteins and a lack of control over cell division, which can lead to breast and/or ovarian cancer. Because they are "autosomal dominant," genetic mutations in BRCA1 and BRCA2 can be passed down to offspring by only one parent, and each child of that carrier has a 50 percent chance of inheriting what journalists have widely (though mistakenly) termed the "breast cancer gene" (Lerner, 276–79). As memoirist Janet Reibstein explains, "It is sometimes said that 'breast cancer genes' have been found. This is not only inaccurate but misleading. . . . Every gene contains a complex set of instructions which normally guide our bodies to work but also can be faulty, giving the wrong information and possibly causing defects and disease. This is what happens in the two 'breast cancer genes' marked so far" (243–44). During the 1990s genetic testing was possible in the United States only through trial studies conducted primarily at academic medical centers, but near the end of the twentieth century it became available commercially through Myriad Genetics. While testing is free in the United Kingdom and Canada through the National Health Service, in the United States it has decreased in cost from as much as $3000 in 2003, depending on whether the test was designed to identify a founder mutation, a single-site mutation, or a full genetic sequencing, to $200 to $300 in 2012. However, as of 2012 genetic testing in the United States was still inconsistently covered by insurance providers (Lerner, 278–79; 23andme. com).

Genetic testing has sometimes been controversial for ethical reasons. Inherited cancers have been found to be especially prevalent among Ashkenazi Jews—studies estimate that one in forty women of this ethnicity carries a BRCA mutation—a fact that has raised the specter of ethnic stereotyping (Lerner, 281–82).[5] In addition, fears of medical and insurance discrimination against people who test positive for genetically triggered diseases abound, although these have been somewhat alleviated by the 2008 passage in the United States of the Genetic Information Nondiscrimination Act (www.facingourrisk.org). While there has been no rush to genetic testing on the part of high-risk women, its commercial availability, along with the suffering that occurs in families who watch loved ones die of breast or ovarian cancer, has led more women than ever before to be tested for BRCA mutations and, if positive, to choose preventive mastectomy. According to the National Cancer Institute, testing has become more widespread in the United States since 2000, and a 2008 study reported in the *Journal of Clinical Oncology* indicates overall satisfaction on the part of women who have undergone prophylactic mastectomy (www.cancer.gov.search/geneticservices; Brandberg, 3943–49).[6] This satisfaction is especially keen among women who had already been diagnosed with cancer in one breast. An October 2007 study in the *Journal of Clinical Oncology* found that the rate of bilateral mastectomies among U.S. women with nonmetastatic breast cancer doubled between 1998 and 2003, from 1.8 to 4.8 percent (Tuttle 5203); of the 78,000 U.S. women who undergo mastectomies each year, researchers estimate that between 8,000 and 10,000 elect prophylactic intervention (Rabin). Since roughly 40,000 U.S. women die each year from breast cancer, these mastectomies are motivated in part by fear; as one woman explained, "You either do it and get on with your life, or you don't, and you risk the possibility of dying" (Springen, 1).

According to Dr. Todd M. Tuttle, chief of surgical oncology at the University of Minnesota Medical Center, several developments are "driving the trend": "More women are going for genetic testing after a diagnosis of breast cancer, and improvements in both mastectomy and breast-reconstruction techniques have made the option of a double reconstruction less daunting" (quoted in Rabin). In some cases women not diagnosed with breast cancer choose preventive mastectomies because they are BRCA-positive and thus have up to an 87 percent risk of contracting the disease if they live into their seventies (Lerner, 279). BRCA-positive women who are pre-menopausal carry especially high risk, and they often experience virulent forms of advanced breast cancer. Prophylactic mastectomy thus provides a potential antidote, since studies suggest that it can lower women's risk by up to 90 percent, depending upon the type of procedure and the amount of tissue removed (Lerner, 286).

Although hundreds of women have been quoted in medical and journalistic articles about prophylactic mastectomy, few have written memoirs that present their genetic histories and medical choices. Those published thus far are by women living in the United States and the United Kingdom, where scientific barriers, cultural prohibitions, and the cost of preventive surgeries have fallen. Memoirs of prophylactic mastectomy juggle autobiographical, educational, and memorializing imperatives, as writers recount their struggles to confront their cancer risk and the surgeries that could minimize that risk, inform readers about the BRCA genetic mutations and the genomic advances of recent decades, and pay elegiac tribute to women in their families who died of genetically driven cancers. Some memoirists employ the military rhetoric decried by Susan Sontag in *Illness as Metaphor*—they wage war against inherited cancers and view prophylactic mastectomies as a means of defeating the enemy— while others describe an existential quest, a wrestling with the fates that would doom them to death by cancer, and posit elective surgery as a way to avoid a "chilly, genetically predestined future" (Queller, 96). Still others approach their cancer legacies pragmatically, accepting available surgical interventions without apparent emotional upheaval.

In this chapter I focus on three compelling postmillennial narratives of prophylactic mastectomy: Janet Reibstein's *Staying Alive: A Family Memoir* (2002), Elizabeth Bryan's *Singing the Life: A Family in the Shadow of Cancer* (2007), and Jessica Queller's *Pretty Is What Changes:*

Impossible Choices, the Breast Cancer Gene, and How I Defied My Destiny (2008). Although Reibstein, Bryan, and Queller tested positive for the BRCA1 genetic mutation, none of them had been diagnosed with breast cancer at the time of her mastectomies; each woman was motivated to undergo surgery by her sense of genetic risk and her painful witness of the death of family members from breast or ovarian cancer. These three writers represent a diversity of ages, nationalities, ethnicities, and professions. Reibstein, an Ashkenazi Jew born in New Jersey, lives in England and works as a psychologist; she was in her late forties in 1995, when her bilateral mastectomy took place, and in her early fifties when she wrote *Staying Alive.* Bryan, an Englishwoman and an Anglican, practiced pediatric medicine in the north of England until her death in 2008; in her late forties she had a preventive oophorectomy, at sixty she underwent a prophylactic double mastectomy, and in her early sixties she wrote her cancer narrative. Queller, also an Ashkenazi Jew, was in her mid-thirties and a New York television writer when she decided in 2005 to undergo a contralateral prophylactic mastectomy and write her family history. All three women are heterosexual, an identity relevant to their narratives because Reibstein and Bryan discuss the effects on their marriages of their decision to undergo preventive mastectomies, while Queller foregrounds her desire to marry and bear children and her initial fear that having prophylactic mastectomies could reduce her chances of finding a male partner. Moreover, as their titles suggest, these writers embrace different narrative foci and generational views: Reibstein emphasizes the quest for survival, having watched her aunts and her mother die of breast cancer; Bryan highlights the importance of celebrating daily life regardless of cancer's shadow; and Queller emphasizes redefined standards of beauty and the urgency of defying destiny.

Despite salient differences, these narratives share three common threads that my analysis seeks to unravel. First, each writer presents an intergenerational account as well as an individual testimony; tales of grandmothers, mothers, aunts, sisters, and cousins figure as prominently as the writer's own story. Thus all three memoirs are haunted by the presence of the dead, as each writer creates a narrative pastiche by including excerpts from her loved ones' journals, letters, and/or poems. Second, each memoirist focuses on three pivotal decisions she must make: whether to be genetically tested; whether, if positive, to undergo mastectomy; and, if so, whether to have reconstructive surgery. Probing the medical, psychological, and sexual considerations that inform these choices constitutes a central imperative in the narratives, and the rhetorical effect is that of a classic bildungsroman, a movement from innocence to experience. Finally, each writer includes a pedagogical postscript in which she probes her post-operative reactions and forges an emotional link to readers by sharing her health-related complications, along with her ethical musings and vision of the future. After analyzing these aspects of the focal narratives I explore briefly the cultural work that they perform, some issues they fail to address, and the competing discourses of self-determination and biological determinism that they feature.

Genealogical Legacies: Cancer as Inheritance

The prologue to Reibstein's narrative depicts her scrutinizing her breasts before the mirror, a pivotal site of both inspection and introspection for many writers of cancer memoirs, and remembering the pleasure those breasts provided during moments of sexual and maternal activity. After bidding them farewell, she affirms her choice to undergo a bilateral prophylactic mastectomy and laments that this option did not exist for her aunts, Fannie Pomerance and Mary Kaufman, or for her mother, Regina Reibstein, each of whom died of metastasized breast cancer—in 1954, 1968, and 1985, respectively. A historical account of the three sisters' immigrant childhoods and the harrowing stories of her aunts' illnesses and demise make up the first third of Reibstein's memoir, while her mother's longer story dominates the middle section; only in the final section does the writer turn to her own experience. This genealogical emphasis occurs through a variety of narrative strategies, most notably Reibstein's graphic depiction of her aunts' mastectomies, invasive follow-up procedures, and painful deaths; and the inclusion of her mother's illness-centered poems and journal entries as a means of memorialization. The result is an elegiac narrative collage, a multigenerational work of cancer auto/biography.

Early in her memoir Reibstein establishes a connection to her Aunt Fannie by describing as her most vivid early childhood memory "the smell of hospitals and with it a picture of myself, bored, looking up at the legs of older relatives hovering around her hospital bed" (39). Diagnosed with breast cancer in 1947 at the age of thirty-three, Fannie had no choice but to undergo a brutal Halsted mastectomy in which "whole chunks of her—a breast and then muscle—were gouged out" (33). In that era, Reibstein reminds readers, this stigmatizing disease was surrounded by silence: "Fannie was one of breast cancer's lonely victims. Women then didn't know that others like them were also fighting in isolation. Young women in particular were hidden—to have a breast full of poison was unspeakable. Fannie would not be able to 'come out' after leaving the hospital" (34). Reibstein further laments the disruptive hormonal treatments her aunt underwent when cancer occurred in Fannie's second breast in 1949, massive radiation to shrink her ovaries and prevent estrogen production, followed by androgen therapy that caused early menopause, masculine features, and behavioral changes: "Her moods swung rapidly and deeply, darkening the world around her and her daughters. She tried to control her temper, but the hormones coursing through her were too powerful" (37). Shortly before her excruciating death, Reibstein explains, Fannie attempted to manipulate her sister Regina's toddler into giving her an overdose of medication; years later, Reibstein's mother wept bitterly when recounting this episode to her writer-daughter. "I can't take any more," Fannie sobbed as Regina confronted her angrily. "He wouldn't have known what he was doing. Who could I ask?" After that episode Fannie disengaged from life, coped with pain only minimally controlled by morphine, and died at forty from bone and spinal metastases (43).

Reibstein's Aunt Mary followed a similar trajectory even though her diagnosis occurred more than a decade later. When she sought treatment in 1967 for a lump in her breast several years after finding it, having decided out of panic to do nothing until it suppurated, Mary endured a Halsted mastectomy followed by massive radiation, an oophorectomy when her ovaries became cancerous, the removal of her pituitary gland to curb estrogen production, and hormonal shifts that changed her appearance and deflated her natural optimism. "In the end Mary became a Fannie," Reibstein asserts, a broken woman who died in isolation, filled with self-hatred and rage (99). By telling her aunts' stories in grim detail Reibstein works against forgetting. In commemorating these women who died before any breast cancer movement, the memoirist pays homage to her matrilineal pioneers and contextualizes her mother's story and her own.

The middle section of Reibstein's narrative shifts focus to her remarkable mother, a poet and community leader who served as president of

New Jersey's League of Women Voters in the 1960s and directed New York's first Commission on the Status of Women in the 1970s. Diagnosed with stage-two breast cancer in 1963 at forty-three, Regina Reibstein also underwent a Halsted mastectomy followed by massive radiation; although she remained healthy for ten years, in 1975 she contracted cancer in her remaining breast and underwent a second mastectomy, further radiation, and chemotherapy, then a new treatment for virulent cancers. Reibstein's genealogical musings continue throughout her account of her mother's saga. During recovery from her first mastectomy, Regina was plagued by memories of Fannie's travails that Reibstein conveys through twin imagery.

> During the days in hospital, awaking to the immediate knowledge that her left breast was gone, that she now had a label, "cancer patient," she'd felt twinned with her dead sister. She ached doubly in her wounds, knowing that Fannie had ached alone. . . . With the realization came guilt. Now, too late, my mother understood the loneliness of Fannie's struggle. (74–75)

Alongside the survivor's guilt of her mother, Reibstein features her own regret at having been in conflict with her mother during her initial illness and recovery. As a high school student reveling in her newfound independence, she resented both her mother's criticism and the inconvenience of her cancer: "I didn't want her to be sick. I was angry at her for being un-whole, vulnerable. Cancer: it was like moral blackmail; I should have been a good person and always borne it in mind. But I couldn't" (89). A painful mother-daughter legacy thus emerges, as Reibstein describes their parallel regret at having disappointed a loved one who suffered from cancer.

Reibstein cements her matrilineal legacy by featuring her mother's writing prominently in her narrative. In 1982, sixty-two years old and in and out of remission from metastatic breast cancer, Regina participated in a University of Chicago–sponsored journal-writing project to document her daily experiences of combating a lethal disease. Reibstein highlights excerpts from her mother's journals as both daughterly tribute and cancer testimony. An entry entitled "Regeneration" from Regina's March 1983 journal, for instance, reflects upon the passive stance she formerly took toward her cancer and her resolve to engage life despite her increasing dependency.

I have had cancer, or more precisely, cancers, for almost twenty
years. My first cancer operation was entirely successful and there
was no metastasis. I was not convinced by medical assurances,
however, and for the next ten years I assumed I was on the verge of
death, suspicious of the least symptom, waiting for the pronounce-
ment, terminal. . . . I no longer cultivate the notion of death. I don't
speculate on which kind of exit appeals most to me. . . . It would not
be so demeaning, I now believe, to accept help and favors. (153–56)

Even as this mother writes philosophically about accepting decline, her
stricken daughter chronicles her own state of denial: given her mother's
accomplishments, Reibstein fantasizes, "maybe she'd be the first to out-
wit advanced breast cancer" (157). The narrative effect of these juxtapositions is a genealogical mirroring: Janet longs futilely for her mother to
survive just as Regina had hoped in vain that her sisters would.

The final matrilineal scene, Regina's farewell visit to Janet just weeks
before her death, portrays what Adrienne Rich in *Of Woman Born* terms
the "mother-daughter cathexis."

The cathexis between mother and daughter—essential, distorted,
misused—is the great unwritten story. Probably there is nothing
in human nature more resonant with charges than the flow of energy between two biologically alike bodies, one of which has lain
in amniotic bliss inside the other, one of which has labored to give
birth to the other. The materials are here for the deepest mutuality
and the most painful estrangement. (226)

Having acknowledged years of estrangement between herself and her
mother, Reibstein represents their last encounter as deeply mutual, an
affirmation driven by grief and familial legacy. When her mother decides
to end her visit early, Reibstein describes her own regression to infancy
and Regina's ultimate act of maternal reassurance.

I felt as if she were literally peeling me off her, like a clinging baby.
But I guess she needed to be on her own to say goodbye to that
wider world which had always drawn her.
On her last night in Cambridge she lay on her bed and cuddled
me as I wept at her leaving. . . . And then out of nowhere she whis-
pered, "I know you think I've always preferred the boys," and she

stroked my hair as if I were small again. . . . "But I haven't. I have loved you as passionately as I've loved them." . . . Everything was healed then. (180)

After her mother's death Reibstein rereads her journals and poems for comfort: "Doing so was a ritual to mutate her into a force inside me, to keep her voice with me. It has worked. I came to feel her as a dispersed presence inside me as I began to build a life in England" (186). What begins as a mourning ritual thus becomes an internalization of her mother's legacy.

Elizabeth Bryan, in *Singing the Life,* also highlights the illness of three sisters, but in her case a genealogical history of ovarian cancer dominates that of breast cancer. The writer's paternal grandmother, her grandfather's sister, and her younger sister, Bernadette (Bunny) Hingley, all died of ovarian cancer, Bryan explains. Shortly before her death in 1995 at forty-seven Bunny tested positive for the BRCA1 genetic mutation, later found to have been passed on through her father. Bryan notes that genetic researchers deemed unusual her family's ovarian cancer history with no comparable history of breast cancer, since the latter disease is usually dominant in carriers of the BRCA1 mutation. Nonetheless, breast cancer had not appeared in Bryan's family until her other sister, Felicity, contracted it in 1999. Bryan incorporates Bunny's and Felicity's illness histories, as well as her cancer genealogy and her own medical saga, through narrative techniques similar to those of Reibstein—the use of family members' journal entries and letters—as well as a second strategy, the inclusion of letters to family members that convey vital medical information.

Early in her narrative Bryan explains that she first learned of her family history through a letter from her father's first cousin, a physician and researcher, who reported "a 50% incidence of ovarian cancer diagnosed in our family on the Hall side in two generations" and urged her female relatives to be vigilant about screening (4). Bryan acknowledges, however, that being thirty-three and healthy she ignored this missive for more than a decade. In 1990, however, unable to have children despite fertility treatments, and past childbearing age, she underwent regular ovarian ultrasound "with a view to having my ovaries removed in the relatively near future" (23). Ironically this decision came just a year before her sister Bunny was diagnosed with lung cancer that had metastasized from the ovaries, a saga that dominates the initial third of Bryan's memoir. The mother of two young daughters and one of England's first female Anglican priests, Bunny documented her cancer in journals from which Bryan quotes extensively. One journal entry recounts Bunny's response to her cancer's recurrence after two years and the terrible prognosis her oncologist offers: "I asked her how I would die, and she said that people died of a blockage in the bowel caused by cancer growth. I asked the final question: how long did she think I had to live? 'I hope you will see the year through,' was the reply" (43). Bryan supplements her sister's journal entries with the disclosure that at Bunny's urging both she and Felicity underwent prophylactic oophorectomies, after which they learned that their ovaries had been healthy.

Bryan intersperses her sister's journal writings with her own account of Bunny's decline, thus assuming the role of familial witness.

> I marveled at how, with the same confidence as she gave her ser-
> mons, but now in pain and heavily drugged with painkillers, she
> dictated fluently the most beautiful and reassuring message to
> each child. . . . For me this was a strange and precious time. Not
> only was I with Bunny, but I was also back in the hospital where
> I had spent my first rewarding and sometimes heart-rending year
> as a doctor. (59–60)

This passage reminds readers that Bryan narrates her family's cancer history not only as a grieving sister but also as a physician for whom any hospital setting is inevitably professional. Nonetheless, her primary narrative impetus is genealogical, as witnessed by her inclusion of elegiac poems written by Bunny's daughter Catherine: "There are too many memories, too many lives, / How will the broken pieces make a whole?" (78).

Bryan's concern for younger generations that must confront their family's genetic history distinguishes her narrative from that of Reibstein, who discusses her two sons' reactions to her cancer but does not highlight next-generation inheritance. Readers meet Bunny's and Felicity's daughters, for whose welfare Bryan assumes medical, ethical, and maternal responsibility, determining not to discuss the family's cancer history until the children reach their twenties. When that time comes Bryan writes them an explanatory letter, included in her narrative, whose tone is straightforward: "As both Felicity and Bunny carried the gene, all four of you have a 50/50 chance of carrying it too. You could all be negative and therefore in the clear. But equally you could all have the bad luck of carrying it" (260). In her narrative reflections Bryan emphasizes the need to let the young make their own confidential decisions regarding genetic testing and preventive surgeries, acknowledging wryly that "for a family who generally talks openly about personal matters this will require restraint from us" (262).

Breast cancer occupies a less central place in Bryan's memoir than in Reibstein's, since Felicity's 1999 diagnosis was the family's first encounter with this disease. Although Felicity, like Bunny, tested positive for BRCA1 after contracting breast cancer, she chose lumpectomy in the hope of preserving her breast; however, radiation and tamoxifen failed to prevent cancer from attacking her other breast, at which time she had a bilateral mastectomy, chemotherapy, and further radiation. Bryan's inclusion of Felicity's 2002 journal entries reinforces her genealogical commitment and introduces new themes such as the militarism of cancer discourse.

> [The surgeon] said that this recurrence showed that my gene was "expressing itself." She need say no more. Without even looking at Alex I looked down at my bosoms and said I regarded them as time bombs and wanted them both off at her earliest convenience. She said that before that she would like me to have other tests to see if the cancer was elsewhere in my body. . . . I saw her point. (99–100)

While Felicity's resilience is moving, her inflated rhetoric of cancerous breasts as "time bombs" is unsettling. After several chapters on Felicity's treatment and recurrence, the narrator foregrounds her own subjectivity: "I felt obliged to think about the future, of the preventive measures I should be considering, and of the next generation" (96).

Jessica Queller focuses in *Pretty Is What Changes* on the death of her mother from ovarian cancer, her own subsequent medical decisions, and those of her younger sister, Danielle. A vexed mother-daughter dynamic dominates the early narrative, as Queller recounts her lifelong ambivalence toward this fashion designer who sported heavy makeup, false eyelashes, and a voluptuous body. Ironically, Stephanie Queller often reminded her daughters they had inherited "good genes," a legacy called into question when she contracted stage-two breast cancer in 1996 and stage-three ovarian cancer in 2002. Queller acknowledges that at the time of her mother's breast cancer their relationship was strained, but the diagnosis caused tensions to ease: "My mother was sick—all else was moot. That said, my mother, sister, and I did not grasp the gravity of breast cancer. The possibility of death was never considered" (33). Instead, the sisters support their mother during grueling chemotherapy treatments while Stephanie worries about hair loss, which, her daughter notes wryly, "to any woman . . . would be a terrible blow, but to my mother was pure horror" (33). Despite her humorous depiction of her mother's vanity, Queller admires this woman who "regardless of nausea, vomiting, mouth sores, or lymphedema . . . exercised on the stairmaster every weekday morning, got dressed in her Armani suits and Manolos, caught the subway, and was in her designer showroom by nine" (34). Using victorious rhetoric that Barbara Ehrenreich views as "denigrating the dead," Queller claims that for years her mother "triumphed over breast cancer" by refusing to see herself as sick (Ehrenreich, 45; Queller, 34–35). She presents her mother's later confrontation with ovarian cancer as similarly embattled but less certain in its outcome: "At age 52, my mother had beaten stage 2 breast cancer. Would this be a harder fight?" (22).

Queller depicts this second cancer as traumatic, for Stephanie loses her hair, her hope, and eventually her life. Still, mother and daughter draw closer during nights Stephanie spends at Jessica's apartment, suffering from chemo's grueling side effects and from terror of death. Queller narrates her despair at her inability to alleviate her mother's suffering, for Stephanie confronts open wounds in her mouth and rectum, a painfully inflamed bowel, and terrible physical disintegration. Like Reibstein, Queller includes in her narrative a deathbed scene in which Stephanie issues delirious commands, whispers to her daughters "I don't want to die," and mutters desperate last words: "Help! This is against my will" (87–89). Although Queller's deathbed narrative offers an anguished immediacy that largely avoids sentimentality, her subsequent reflection on matrilineal inheritance does become sentimental: "As her illness progressed and she became increasingly present as a mother, my judgments against the material things she loved were silenced. Now, every item that belonged to my mom was endowed with emotion. . . . I'd begun wearing her heels to work. As I traipsed up the stairs to join the other writers, I realized I was literally and metaphorically walking in my mother's shoes" (90–91).

Although Queller does not incorporate her mother's writing into her narrative, as do Reibstein and Bryan, she includes a letter of tribute from a woman who met Stephanie when the two were receiving post-operative

treatment at the same hospital. Queller uses this letter to enhance readers' understanding of her mother's illness experience and to foreground
breast cancer sisterhood, even when the women are apolitical. "I had just
turned forty and my third son was twelve months old," the friend, Liza
Wherry, explains.

> Your mother was fifty. Right away we liked one another and we
> were the first "breast cancer friends" one another had come into
> contact with in the days following our surgeries. Also, I am not a
> "political breast cancer patient." I don't go on marches and don't
> seek out other women who had had breast cancer. I don't wear a
> pink baseball cap and a Susan Komen t-shirt. It just isn't me. I got
> the feeling that your mother, too, (as we stood outside Dr. Roses'
> office waiting for him to arrive) was a more discreet person and
> not one to devote her life to being a "survivor" (a word I really
> don't like). (163)

In subsequent encounters, the letter continues, Liza and Stephanie shared
agitation over chemotherapy, laughed at Liza's expensive wig in the hospital restroom, and comforted one another. Wherry's letter confirms
Queller's belief that her ill mother became "more maternal": "In many
of our phone calls your mother indicated how concerned she was about
her 'girls' . . . she didn't want you and your sister to worry nor have added
stress in your lives" (165). The inclusion of this letter adds emotional heft
to Queller's memoir, while its content affirms a matrilineal bond.

Their genealogical memoirs reveal Reibstein, Bryan, and Queller as
haunted by ghostly revenants, the women in their families who died of
cancer but inspire the living to survive it. Commemorative, informa-
tional, and autobiographical impulses intersect, as each writer carries
memories of her aunts, mothers, and/or sisters to the printed page.

Vexed Decisions: Genetic Testing, Preventive Surgery,
Breast Reconstruction

According to their memoirs, the decision of whether to be tested for a
BRCA genetic mutation was easy for all three of these writers to make,
but for different reasons. For Bryan it was pro forma: given her curiosity as a physician, her family history of ovarian cancer, and her sister's

death, she never doubted that she would seek testing once commercial procedures became available. In 1999 she learned from a Cambridge genetic researcher who had been studying her family's history through the United Kingdom's Familial Ovarian Cancer Register that his team had identified a "pathogenic mutation" in the BRCA1 gene, "a deletion of 4 bases designated 3875 del 4," as the cause of the high incidence of ovarian cancer in her family; he urged Bryan to undergo genetic testing so that her risk could be quantified (92). Having taken the test, Bryan felt "a rather weary acceptance" upon learning that she had inherited the mutation (93). Since she had already undergone a prophylactic oophorectomy, she considered that decision vindicated by the research findings but was not concerned about her breast cancer risk because at that point no family member had ever been stricken. Several months later, however, her sister Felicity learned that she had breast cancer, and shortly afterward Bryan tested positive for BRCA1 (94).

As a woman in her thirties, Queller belongs to a generation that views genetic testing as simply a facet of modern life. She explains in her memoir that she neither remembers a time when this procedure was unavailable nor considers it ethically vexed. Yet taking a genetic test was for her precautionary; never did she imagine that her mother's cancer might have been genetically triggered.

> I wanted to take the test simply for the peace of mind of having a clean bill of health in writing. . . . In spite of the fact that my mother had cancer twice, I did not feel the disease would ever strike me. I had witnessed the horror of cancer up-close. I knew my mother had been shocked each time she'd been seized by cancer. And yet, strangely, I still felt invincible. (92)

When she learned her results in 2004, Queller felt ill-prepared to cope with being BRCA-positive or with the doctor's claim that she would have an 85–90 percent chance of contracting breast cancer in her lifetime, information that stunned her even as she suspected that it would change her life.

Reibstein reports having initially decided not to be genetically tested because of her confidence that she would test positive, given her family history and her cousin Joyce's recent contraction of cancer in both breasts. Rather than seek testing she undergoes a bilateral prophylactic mastectomy, yet despite her certainty she is shocked to learn that her amputated breast tissue contains multiple sites of carcinoma in situ, a precancerous condition whose traces indicate that she likely carries the mutation: "We daughters of breast cancer mothers were thinking: maybe not us. Maybe our mothers' deaths were a fluke of their Paterson childhood. Maybe the cancers were entirely environmentally caused. Maybe no faulty genes were involved at all" (188). In her narrative Reibstein acknowledges the depths to which denial can extend in women with familial cancer histories.

For each narrator an especially vexed decision was whether to remove her apparently healthy breasts. Bryan records the least angst, although for two years after testing BRCA-positive she underwent frequent screening rather than taking more drastic measures, but motivated by her sister's breast cancer recurrence, she determined at last "to be rid of my potentially deadly appendages" (103). Her concern that "it seemed heartless to be thinking of removing two healthy breasts when she [Felicity] had no option but to suffer the physical and emotional trauma of losing hers to cancer" was mitigated when her sister urged Bryan to undergo prophylactic mastectomies (104). As suggested by her use of the word *appendages,* Bryan acknowledges that breasts were not important to her body image and that she harbored no nostalgic memories of breastfeeding. Instead she wanted to stay alive—for her pediatric work, for her husband, a cancer survivor himself, and for the next generation. Sexuality was not a factor in her decision: "Even without the setbacks, at 60 and 74 I doubt that our sex life would have been a page-turner. Indeed it probably never had been. Sex had always been a very happy, straightforward, vital and yet unadventurous part of our life" (111). While acknowledging women who fear that removing healthy breasts might compromise their femininity, Bryan explains that she felt differently: "my breasts were not something for which I had a particular affection" (103). Aware that preventive surgery would not be covered under NHS, her primary concern was choosing an experienced private surgeon who would respect her decision and answer her questions fully. Having done so, in November 2002 she underwent a bilateral prophylactic mastectomy.

Reibstein describes her decision as more complicated, in part because her process began in 1990, when taboos were greater and post-operative silence reigned.

A small but growing number of women in the U.S. had chosen this operation. However, the sisterhood of prophylactic mastectomy survivors was secret. People remained revolted and confused by the notion that a woman would willingly undergo mastectomy without a definite diagnosis of breast cancer. Women with breast cancer had come out of the shadows, but what was done to them hadn't. . . . Albeit no longer "dirty" or the death of a women's sexuality, [mastectomy] remained horrid and hidden because it might signal death. (203–4)

This passage reminds readers of the cultural shifts during the two past decades in breast cancer awareness and of the isolation experienced by many pioneers of prophylactic mastectomy. Reibstein records the outrage she feels at the reactions of others: "Some friends were terribly shocked, even repelled, by my decision. That was much as I'd expected, but it angered me. For God's sake, what are a pair of breasts worth compared to survival?" (207). She further explains that over the years she had begun to question the cultural fetishizing of cleavage and eventually "came to dislike breasts in general, and mine in particular" (193). Yet only when her cousin contracted cancer in her second breast did Reibstein decide to act, and only on the gurney did she realize the significance of her decision.

What I was about to do represented the cutting edge (literally) of what women with an inherited tendency towards breast cancer could do to prevent it. Not great, perhaps, and possibly not what would be done ten, twenty, thirty years from now, but so much better than waiting for the probable diagnosis one day. My operation also signified amazing progress for a far larger population than the relatively few of us with a wonky genetic loading. (212)

Queller expresses anguish about prophylactic mastectomy because of her youth and her concerns about sexuality. Following confirmation by phone that she had tested positive for BRCA1, she describes receiving an ominous report by mail.

In the center of the report: POSITIVE FOR A DELETERIOUS MUTATION was printed in bold letters and framed by a rectangular box for emphasis. The paragraph underneath contained the grim statistics the doctor had told me over the phone, but in greater detail: "Deleterious mutations in BRCA1 may confer as much as an 87% risk of breast cancer and a 44% risk of ovarian cancer by age 70 in women. Mutations in BRCA1 have been reported to confer a 20% risk of a second breast cancer within five years of the first as well as a ten-fold increase in the risk of subsequent ovarian cancer." (96)

This information underscores the pedagogical imperative of Queller's narrative, which urges readers to learn about genetic risks. Still, she too acknowledges having engaged in denial for months before seeking genetic counseling, and she admits feeling anger at her counselor's suggestion that she consider having prophylactic surgery. "Was she out of her mind?" Queller wonders on her drive home, dismayed by the chilling Ca 125 blood test to which she had been subjected, the "claustrophobic, loud and eerie" MRI, and the sonogram that led doctors to palpitate her fibrocystic breasts (102). "Back off," she instructs her friend Kay, who urges Queller to consider the geneticist's advice: "There was no way I was going to *cut my breasts off*" (104).

A professional opportunity causes Queller to reconsider prophylactic mastectomy: an invitation to write an op-ed column for the *New York Times* about testing positive for the BRCA1 mutation. By her own admission Queller led a privileged life: a highly paid writer for the television series *The Gilmore Girls,* she jetted weekly between New York and Los Angeles and encountered celebrities daily at her Hollywood studio office. Hoping that a column in the *Times* would advance her journalistic career, she began the research into breast cancer genetics that would later inform her decision about preventive mastectomy. The publication of her *New York Times* article provoked a family conflict: the evening before the column appeared, Queller reports, her sister expressed anger at being "outed" as a member of a cancer-prone family: "Your taking the test has cancelled out my choice to remain sheltered from all of this. And your writing about it has taken away my privacy" (155). Stunned and apologetic, Queller realizes that in making her own medical decision she has overlooked her sister's right to privacy. Although the narrative never probes this issue in depth, Queller, like Bryan, raises in her memoir the important topic of ethical accountability.

As someone whose family history included not only breast and ovarian cancer but also an emphasis on bodily perfection, Queller writes frankly of the psychological struggle her consideration of prophylactic mastectomy evoked. Uncomfortable with her large breasts and with the cultural sexualization of women, she nonetheless admits, "I had a love-hate relationship with my breasts. I did not want to be valued for them. . . . At the same time I understood that men found my body sexy and I liked that" (124). Concerned that her sex life would suffer if she had surgery, Queller poses a series of questions that reveal the gender-essentialist perspective that dominates her narrative: "Would men no longer find me desirable? Would I feel deformed? Would I ever want to be touched again? Would I no longer feel like a whole woman?" (127). In addition to these fears, she acknowledges wanting a child and, at thirty-five and single, feeling "already up against the biological clock" (128). Despite her worries, Queller describes an epiphany she experienced during an interview with Cokie Roberts on *Nightline.* "Having watched my mother die a brutal, horrific death," she tells Roberts, "I would do anything" to avoid dying of cancer (187). On a vacation shortly before her surgery, Queller affirms her decision in a journal entry: "Having surgery is taking care of myself. My true self. My spirit, my character, stuff on the inside. Whatever the cosmetic result of my body, my breasts, is not all that consequential" (221). Thus in September 2005 she underwent a prophylactic mastectomy performed by the same surgeon who had operated on her mother years earlier. Queller's account of the night before her surgery employs war imagery to presents her journey as bildungsroman: "I felt remarkably calm. I was ready for battle. . . . I thought of what I was about to endure as a rite of passage into adulthood" (228). Like Reibstein, Queller views her post-operative pathology report as vindicating this decision, since it revealed atypical ductal hyperplasia, pre-cancerous tissue, in her right breast. "You did the right thing," her surgeon assures her (234).

These writers also detail the reasons they choose breast reconstruction. Bryan offers a familial justification: to protect her young nieces, with whom she often shared a room when vacationing, from seeing their aunt's post-operative chest and learning too early of their genetic legacy. She explains to readers her decision to have silicone implant reconstruction at the time of her mastectomies, with the understanding that nipples would later be tattooed on or rebuilt from skin. Although she never expresses regret, Bryan acknowledges that reconstruction entailed "a higher price to pay in worry, money and discomfort than I had expected" (105). A gruesome saga follows, as she describes her leaky, swollen left breast, infected a week after surgery, its failure to respond to antibiotics, and the subsequent removal of her implant, a procedure that left her asymmetrical and in pain. She further records her surprise at how "ugly" she found artificial breasts without nipples ("they badly need adornment"), her humorous efforts to recall the tint of her original nipples so that the prosthetic ones could match, and her relief when the reconstructive process was completed: "I felt transformed" (111).

Both Reibstein and Queller decide upon reconstructive surgery only after viewing the post-operative breasts of other women. Reibstein notes in her narrative that she experienced these encounters as traumatic. "It took me two years to talk to the two survivors. To do so represented a major step towards my decision. If I talked to them I was facing it. I knew I wouldn't retreat from what they'd tell me, and I knew that what they'd tell me was that they did not regret their surgery" (193). When she finally views an acquaintance's reconstructed breasts, the narrator describes both appreciation and shock at the scars, surgical nipples, and unconvincing breasts she confronted: "I went white when she showed me hers; I hadn't really registered that I would indeed look different from the way I'd always looked—how could I when there were no pictures? I'd even nurtured a fantasy my breasts would be improved—the sag lifted, the size perfect" (206). Although she hid her negative reaction, Reibstein admits that she later "had vivid dreams about ugly and distended bodies, bodies mutilated" and that only in retrospect did she appreciate the value of knowing what her new breasts might look like (207). Queller, in contrast, is inspired by her encounter with a friend who underwent prophylactic mastectomies and reconstruction; she views this woman's reconstructed breasts as "rather beautiful" and "astonishingly real" (150).

Surgical reconstruction becomes problematic for Reibstein but is largely positive for Queller, as each explains in her memoir. Throughout 1994, Reibstein discussed reconstructive options with her surgeon and finally selected a subcutaneous mastectomy that would preserve her nipple, allow soy implants to be inserted, but remove only 90 percent of her breast tissue, thus leaving a potential site for further exposure to cancer. She rues this decision when her surgeon finds carcinoma in situ in both breasts and recommends another surgery to remove the remaining tissue. Reibstein details the infections, medical complications, and additional surgeries that led ultimately to the removal of her soy implants and the implantation of silicone alternatives. In contrast, Queller recounts a largely successful reconstructive process. Although fluid accumulation and leakage require antibiotics and extensive drainage, she is ultimately pleased with the feel of her silicone implants, the natural appearance of her nipples, and the size she chooses for her new breasts: 32B rather than the 32D's toward which she had long felt ambivalent. Her decision to reduce her breast size signifies a rejection of cultural sexualization and a fulfillment of her desire for agency in constructing her own hybrid body.

In their narrative accounts of genetic testing, preventive mastectomy, and breast reconstruction, these memoirists grapple with questions of sexuality, identity, and medical efficacy: What effects does a prophylactic mastectomy have on the patient's sexuality? How does it affect her sense of self, of wholeness?[7] What medical risks accompany such surgeries, how effective are they in preventing breast cancer, and which types of procedure retain valuable chest muscle and tissue while minimizing risk of cancer occurring there? Ultimately each writer expresses confidence in her decision to be genetically tested, choose preventive mastectomy, and undergo breast reconstruction.

Postscripts / Cautionary Tales / Future Visions

In Reibstein's final chapter readers find her sunbathing in 1999 on a Mediterranean beach, wearing an old red bathing suit and pondering her new body: "I like my shape. These breasts are neither beautiful nor grotesque. They are neither me nor not me" (238). She further recognizes, as she surveys the topless women around her, that breasts no longer serve as markers of beauty or desirability—that she is "beyond breasts" (239). This realization comes, however, after major complications from multiple reconstructive surgeries, from life-threatening infections to implant removal to disfiguring scars, which she recounts in her postscript. Reibstein further reflects upon the phenomenon of many Western women now living with advanced breast cancer rather than dying from it. While she has prevented cancer by choosing prophylactic surgery, she describes many friends with chronic breast cancer who "lead comfortable lives, their periods of medical treatment relatively short and compassionate, despite inevitable suffering and discomfort, in comparison to what Regina, Mary, and Fannie endured twenty, thirty, and fifty years ago" (243). Pleased that "knowledge of the genetics of breast cancer has exploded," she explains how a family genogram finally confirmed that she carries the BRCA1 mutation, probably passed down from her mother's father (243–45). Reibstein's conclusion exudes optimism: genetic consultations are readily available in the twenty-first century; prophylactic mastectomies for BRCA-positive women save lives; and she is thrilled to consider herself cured. Her final paragraph returns to the genealogical reflection with which her narrative began, but with a triumphant tone previously absent.

> I went one better than my mother. Because of her I fought. Because of her I was vigilant. Because I live when I do, I stopped it, caught it quickly, and survived. . . . I know she would be proud of me. I have imagined her loving me through this very strongly. I can almost see her crowing down from an imaginary Heaven, shouting "That's my girl!" It would be great if the next generation could go on to be free of the shadow, free, too, of the knife. Now *that* my mother, and her sisters, would have loved. (248)

Despite her problematic use of triumphalist rhetoric, Reibstein's conclusion remains compelling because it envisions increasing numbers of women free of cancer's shadow.[8]

As a physician Bryan makes an overt pedagogical commitment to readers by including appendices that describe the BRCA1 mutation in lay language, assess the ethical and medical questions raised by genetic testing and elective surgeries, and define key terms used in the narrative. Especially informative is a concluding chapter, "BRCA1 Today and Our Family," which notes that in 2006 the Human Fertilization and Embryology Authority in the United Kingdom endorsed pre-implantation genetic diagnosis, or PGD for the BRCA1 and BRCA2 gene mutations, and explains that PGD enables carriers who wish to have children to engage in an in vitro fertilization procedure that tests the cells of embryos, to implant a BRCA-negative embryo, and thereby to avoid passing on the mutation to their fetus. She probes the ethical implications of this procedure by presenting differing views of medical practitioners and her own family members and by acknowledging relief that she did not have to make such a vexing decision.

Bryan's narrative conclusion jolts readers by revealing her diagnosis at sixty-three of advanced pancreatic cancer, after which she undergoes surgery and chemotherapy. Given this cancer's virulence, she experiences a recurrence one year after her original diagnosis and acknowledges in her memoir that she is dying as she writes; her narrative thus shifts from autopathography to autothanatography. Nonetheless, she continues to chronicle her disease dispassionately, explaining that while breast cancer represents 23 percent of all cancers in women, pancreatic cancer represents only 3 percent; that the lifetime risk of contracting breast cancer is 1 in 9 for women in England, while the risk of pancreatic cancer is 1 in 95; that only 13 percent of patients with pancreatic cancer survive more than a year after diagnosis and 2–3 percent more than five years; and that while she hopes to be one of the survivors, she does not expect to be (160–61). Curiosity leads her to investigate whether her BRCA1 status might have been a factor in causing her pancreatic cancer, a determination she ultimately deems impossible to make, and she describes her excitement at being one of the two first pancreatic cancer patients to enter a trial study to assess potential links to BRCA1 and her later disappointment that the trial medications worsen her cancer and necessitate her withdrawal from the study. Through all of this Bryan remains philosophical: while she acknowledges that prophylactic surgery might have led her BRCA mutation to manifest in the pancreas because less deadly locations were no longer available, she refuses to dwell on that possibility, admitting merely that she feels "a bit miffed" to have undergone prophylactic mastectomies only to contract a more virulent cancer (293). In the final pages readers witness Bryan's physical decline and preparation for death, as she shares farewell emails sent to family and friends, and describes her participation in a gathering of music and tributes that she considers a prelude to her own funeral. In "A Husband's Afterword" readers learn that Bryan died peacefully at home in February 2008; her final words were "wonderful, wonderful" (294). Bryan's narrative violates readers' expectations by ending not with the recovery of the narrator but with her untimely death. *Singing the Life* thus serves as authorial self-commemoration as well as a narrative of intergenerational genetic cancers.

In the postscript to *Pretty Is What Changes* Queller extends her matrilineal emphasis, reveals her experience of post-operative sexuality, and establishes her identity as a cancer activist. She chronicles her sister Danielle's decision to undergo a prophylactic double mastectomy in 2007, motivated not only by Jessica's act but also by the discovery of their mother's breast cancer journal, which she interpreted as a sign: "Our mother was speaking directly to her from beyond the grave . . . telling her to have the operation and have it now" (265). A year earlier, Queller explains, Danielle had tested positive for the BRCA1 mutation; that discovery and her decision to have surgery had strengthened the sisters' bond. Queller also discusses her embrace of breast cancer activism as a *previvor*—a term for BRCA-positive women who choose preventive surgery—who has joined

FORCE (Facing Our Risk of Cancer Empowered), a U.S. organization for women at risk for genetically driven cancers. She further reports that she and her sister received the Lynne Cohen Foundation's 2007 "Courageous Spirit Award" for testifying publicly about their prophylactic mastectomies.

Queller's narrative concludes with the news that single, thirty-seven, and eager to have a child, she is "heading to the sperm bank" (273). As part of in vitro fertilization she plans to take a PGD test that will allow her to select for uterine implantation an embryo that does not carry the BRCA1 mutation, thus assuring a genetic erasure of her familial cancer history. An important aspect of Queller's postscript is her ethical reflection on PGD testing.

> Had this technology been available in 1969, I would have ended up in the trash can. Can I, in good faith, choose embryos that don't have the mutation and destroy the others? Is taking action to ensure my unborn child will not have to go through the terrors my mother, sister, and I have suffered the responsible choice? Or is it immoral to extinguish a life merely because it carries a gene that I myself live with? (274)

She ponders how far U.S. society will and should go to engineer embryos and what new technological options stem cell research might produce. Moral and pedagogical imperatives converge as Queller expresses her belief in "utilizing biotechnology to promote health," extols the scientific opportunities now available to save lives, and urges readers to "seize them" (274, 277).

Environmental Myopia and Competing Discourses

What do narratives of prophylactic mastectomy contribute to their readers' understanding of the breast cancer continuum? What do such narratives offer as postmillennial cultural commentary? For women considering genetic testing or preventive surgery, these narratives provide information and possibly inspiration. For academic and general readers they offer new medical and technological knowledge as well as riveting autobiographical profiles. Any remaining social stigma attached to the choice of prophylactic mastectomy for women who test positive for

BRCA1 or BRCA2 can arguably be lessened by such memoirs; new affiliations can be established between women who have entered the "uncharted waters" of our DNA age and readers who bear witness to their journeys (Queller, 274).

While I applaud these writers for raising awareness about genetically inherited cancers, I share the concern of Eisenstein in *Manmade Breast Cancers* that environmental factors are downplayed in assessments of genetic cancers, and I find such minimizing troubling in the prophylactic mastectomy narratives under consideration.[9] Eisenstein argues that breast cancer must be seen as "a social and political/biological problem defined by the food and tobacco industry, the military-industrial complex, and corporate polluters" (78). Indeed, the breast itself requires reimagining, and she offers a template for doing so.

> Connect it to the body systematically and to its complex environments cyclically. Define our environments with open yet connected boundaries between air, water, soil, economic and racial hierarchies, and the female body.
>
> Interrogate the cause/effect scientific model for its linear blinders. Supplant this model with an interactive and multistage model of malignant growth that recognizes the interstices between bodies, genes, and environments. (76)

Although such a template might reasonably be viewed as the work of medical researchers rather than memoirists, I wished for more consideration of intersections between genetic and environmental cancer influences in the narratives of Bryan, Reibstein, and Queller.

To be sure, Bryan and Reibstein acknowledge that environmental factors might play a role in determining which BRCA-positive women will contract breast and/or ovarian cancer, but they largely embrace a single-causality approach. Bryan correctly points out that "environmental influences, including diet, can influence the appearance of a cancer even when it is primarily determined by one's genes" and that it is "not yet understood why some people who carry the BRCA1 cancer gene survive into old age with no sign of cancer while the majority show it much earlier in life" (154). She does not, however, explore the role that environmental toxins play in causing cancer to manifest. Reibstein goes further, noting that "carcinogens are multiplying in the environment, due to industrial processes, vehicle emissions, factory farming, food technology and packaging" and that "this greater load of carcinogenic pollutants presumably increases the probability of cancer being triggered earlier" (241). Still, she fails to assign to these carcinogens a greater causal significance than diet, longevity, and lifestyle, and she views genetic mutation as the greatest risk factor (241). Queller barely mentions environmental links to BRCA-related cancers, noting merely that her research provided "no medical consensus on what factors caused expression of the gene," although she mentions diet, reproductive history, and "environmental exposures" as possible factors (119). Overall, environmental carcinogens receive minimal emphasis in genetically centered sagas.

These narratives rely instead on discourses of biological determinism that assume the veracity of the adage "biology is destiny" even as they laud new biotechnologies. Queller's subtitle, "How I Defied My Destiny," best exemplifies this discursive tendency, but Bryan exhibits it as well by endorsing the view that her sister has contracted breast cancer because "her gene [was] expressing itself," despite the fact no other BRCA-positive family members had ever had breast cancer (99). Reibstein comes closest to recognizing Eisenstein's perspective that genetics is but one potential factor in causing breast cancer, since she acknowledges that in future studies BRCA status might "have more muted roles in cancerous growth than we think," but she offers no further consideration of breast cancer's environmental links (244). In addition, discourses of self-determination often compete in these narratives with discourses of genetic absolutism. Reibstein and Queller, in particular, boast of conquering or outwitting breast cancer through canny use of biotechnological advances and willpower: Reibstein claims to have "defeated the thing" her mother merely strove to conquer (248), while Queller describes having "decided to live," as if Bryan and other women who lost their lives to cancer decided to die (book cover). Although readers can appreciate these narratives of prophylactic mastectomy for their autobiographical, pedagogical, and commemorative power, it is important from a feminist perspective to query their problematic representation of genes as destiny to be defied through an unsettling combination of self-aggrandizing agency and cutting-edge biotechnologies available to many wealthy women of the world, but certainly not to all.

4 | Rebellious Humor in Breast Cancer Narratives
Deflating the Culture of Optimism

way to cope

Despite the seriousness of the disease, not all breast cancer narratives are somber; many are actually funny. Indeed, rebellious humor serves as an antidote to resignation and despair in postmillennial autobiographical writing by scores of U.S. women about their cancer experience, from diagnosis to surgery to chemotherapy and/or radiation to recovery and/or recurrence. My informal November 2008 survey of 210 books and items for sale on amazon.com under the heading "breast cancer products" revealed that more than half employ humor as a dominant motif, as seen in such titles as *Five Lessons I Didn't Learn from Cancer* by Shelley Lewis, *Cancer Is a Bitch* by Gail Konop Baker, *Just Get Me Through This!* by Deborah A. Cohen and Robert M. Gelfand, *It's Not About the Hair* by Debra Jarvis, and *Crazy Sexy Cancer Tips* by Kris Carr. In addition, cynical surveyors of the amazon.com list might find humor that authors do not intend in such titles as *Pink Prayer, Chicken Soup for the Breast Cancer Survivor's Soul,* and *Kitchen Aid Cook for the Cure,* whose cover features a pink mixer and measuring spoons, also for sale. During National Breast Cancer Awareness Month (NBCAM) in October 2008 Lifetime Television aired several made-for-TV films with humorous or tragicomic breast cancer themes, including a *Sex in the City*–style comedy produced by Renée Zellweger based on journalist Geralyn Lucas's memoir *Why I Wore Lipstick to My Mastectomy.* A recent google.com search using the heading "breast cancer humor" produced a staggering 1,640,000 links, and a brief trek through only 200 of them led to such diverse websites as www.boycottoctober.com, www.cancerplanet.com, and www.thecancerblog.com, as well as organizational websites from www.breastcancer.org to www.komen.org to www.bcaction.org.

To understand how and why rebellious humor is central to many women's cancer experience, and to their written accounts of that experience, it is useful to extrapolate from Jo Anna Isaak's analysis of "primary narcissism" in the self-portraits of two late twentieth-century photographers who died of the disease, Jo Spence and Hannah Wilke. Each artist chronicled her decline photographically—medicalized, bald, naked, dying, *and* laughing, sometimes heartily, sometimes grimly. Isaak's argument about the power of these photographs stems in part from Freud's assertions in his 1927 essay "On Humour."

> *Humour is not resigned; it is rebellious* . . . It also has something of grandeur and elevation. . . . The grandeur in it clearly lies in *the triumph of narcissism,* the victorious assertion of the ego's invulnerability. The ego refuses to be distressed by the provocations of reality, to let itself be compelled to suffer. It insists that it cannot be affected by the traumas of the external world; it shows, in fact, that such traumas are no more than the occasions for it to gain pleasure. (162–63)   ⟶ couℓd be useful

Isaak rightly critiques Freud's sexism as revealed in an earlier essay, "On Narcissism," in which he claims that women in particular exhibit narcissistic behaviors, thereby engaging what she describes as "a lost state of self-sufficiency that the male has relinquished" (Freud, 89; Isaak, 53). Yet she notes that Freud does not decry narcissism when he associates it with defiant humor, which can lead to empowering forms of agency. Isaak views women photographers' strategic use of narcissism in their cancer self-portraits as a performative act, "a site of pleasure and a form of resistance to assigned sexual and social roles" that would posit ill women as victims and conceal their dying bodies (54). Spence and Wilke thus find pleasure in challenging both misogyny and medicalization through their cancer photographs. Bare-breasted to reveal her lumpectomy scar in *The Picture of Health?* Spence dons a helmet to signify resistance to hegemonic medical practices and to ridicule machismo. In her *Intra-Venus* series Wilke puns on the word *intravenous;* in one photograph she is nude, taped up for chemotherapy, and balancing a flower arrangement on her head to parody hegemonic femininity.[1] Isaak rightly concludes that "in assuming the role of the clown in the face of death," Spence and Wilke "take this humor through annihilation—humor is the attack, the dissolution of the ego and the subject" (66).

My assessment of postmillennial memoirists' use of breast cancer humor reveals their reliance on transgressive textual strategies that help them confront as vibrant, laughing subjects (not as abject objects) the vulnerabilities that accompany a life-threatening disease. Even when the writer does not so identify herself, rebellious humor seems feminist in its resistant consciousness. In a culture that obsessively sexualizes women's breasts, that professes to revere the nursing mother (even if the reality of women breast-feeding in public remains off-putting for many), and that views thick, glossy hair as a quintessential feminine feature, mastectomy, lumpectomy, and hair loss during chemo might well threaten the gendered identity (as distinct from the hegemonic femininity) of even the most ardent feminist. For this reason, the travails of pre- and post-surgical breasts and the baldness of "wigged out" cancer patients are among the most prevalent subjects of women's humorous memoirs, along with the grueling side effects of cancer treatment: nausea, weight gain or loss, waning sexual desire, physical exhaustion, and the mental impairment known informally as "chemo brain."[22] Other recurring comic themes include the alienating machines and procedures that patients encounter during their diagnoses and surgeries, the actions and temperaments of medical practitioners, the inappropriate responses of well-meaning family members and friends, the blame-the-victim mentality that dies hard in U.S. culture, and the self-help and alternative medicine industries that recommend as antidotes to cancer everything from yoga to visualization to group therapy. For writers for whom survival seems unlikely, the use of "humor through annihilation" produces ironic accounts of their shocking metastases and virulent follow-up treatments (Isaak, 60).

Postmillennial breast cancer memoirists employ three strategies of representation to convey their humorous (and sometimes tragicomic) tropes: self-deprecation, self-division, and self-assertion. Self-deprecation offers a subversive challenge to what Isaak calls the "masquerade of femininity" (67). By approaching breast cancer through the guise of a woman proudly lacking in hyperfemininity, memoirists adopt a performative stance designed to evoke the reader's laughter through identification with body-centered foibles and fears. Self-division is used by cancer humorists to ironize dualism and incongruity, long identified as sources of classic comedy. As Isaak points out, Freud's "On Humour" was influenced by Baudelaire's 1855 essay "On the Essence of Laughter," which posits that laughter "belongs to the class of all artistic phenomena that show the existence in the human being of a permanent dualism, the capacity of being oneself and someone else at the same time" (Baudelaire, 160). For many cancer memoirists, an especially funny subject is human incongruity, an uneasy doubling often manifested in strategic dual personae. "*I* don't have breast cancer (or nausea or a bald head or chemo brain)," this rubric of displacement implies, "*that woman does.*" Like self-deprecation, the divided self is often an emotional reality for these writers and a theatrical tactic, and the laughter that it generates thus becomes "diabolic in nature, both a symptom of loss and division and the means of redemption" (Isaak, 54). And self-assertion provides writers of humorous breast cancer narratives with a sense of boundlessness, for as Freud noted, "humour has something liberating about it" ("On Humour," 162).   ↳ humor can be freeing

Humorous breast cancer memoirs also have sociopolitical dimensions. A frequent subject of critique is the survivor discourse encouraged by advocacy groups from the American Cancer Society to Susan G. Komen Race for the Cure. Narratives that interrogate NBCAM, for example, raise readers' consciousnesses along with revealing the writers' cultural misgivings about corporate disease philanthropy; they employ satire and self-assertion to dissect the breast cancer marketplace. In addition, many comic memoirists rebel against breast cancer culture's tyrannical cheerfulness, as exhibited in discourses that highlight blissful survivors whose lives have improved dramatically and that criticize women who express anger or fear. While humor is a dominant strategy, few of these memoirists participate in the mass-produced optimism that characterizes mainstream cancer organization websites and brochures; they prefer a postmodern sense of contingency that deflects rather than embraces sentimental discourses.

In this chapter I analyze three types of humorous breast cancer memoirs: personal narratives that use linear retrospection to present their confrontation with this life-threatening illness, illustrated here by Meredith Norton's *Lopsided: How Having Breast Cancer Can Be Really Distracting* (2008); graphic narrative depictions of the breast cancer continuum, represented here by Miriam Engelberg's *Cancer Made Me a Shallower Person: A Memoir in Comics* (2006); and memoirs that began as blogs, illustrated here by S. L. Wisenberg's *The Adventures of Cancer Bitch* (2009). These writers reflect diverse generations, ethnicities, and professions: Norton, an African American woman living in France, was thirty-four years old and the at-home mother of an infant son when diagnosed with inflammatory breast cancer; Engelberg, an Ashkenazi Jew, was forty-three and a professional cartoonist at the time her advanced breast cancer was discovered; and Wisenberg, also Jewish American, was a university professor in her fifties at the time of diagnosis. Regardless of whether their chosen form is linear retrospection, sequential art, or blog-cum-memoir, these postmillennial mammographers use breast cancer humor to defy their disease's destructive power, question invasive medical interventions, and undermine the pieties of cancer culture.

Self-Deprecation and Cultural Critique in *Lopsided*

When Meredith Norton realized something was wrong with her breast, she was a nursing mother living in Paris—homesick, alienated from French culture, and frustrated by inadequate medical care. Having noticed that her breasts had become "comically askew," she initially attributed this change to the perils of lactation.

> Lactating breasts behave oddly. . . . One of mine was huge, throbbing, covered with a red rash, and radiating enough heat to defrost a frozen lamb shank in ten minutes. It was like an unpredictable little alien I carried around. Even in the kooky world of milk-making tits, this one worried me. (16)

When she stopped breast-feeding her year-old son, Lucas, her engorged breast remained so painful that she sought medical assistance, but receiving no help from four French physicians, whose recommendations ranged from a "waxy poultice" to antibiotics, Norton decides to return to California, take Lucas to visit "his loud, Black American family," and "maybe see a real doctor about my boob" (17). These quotations illustrate Norton's primary strategies for inducing her readers' laughter: exaggeration combined with graphic imagery, a blunt interrogation of the Otherness that Blackness often signifies and illness intensifies, a satiric approach to unappetizing medical treatment, and a colloquial discourse of tits, boobs, and kookiness.

Diagnosed with stage-three inflammatory breast cancer that required chemotherapy, mastectomy, then radiation, and told by her consulting physicians that she had a 40 percent chance of surviving five years, Norton responds with numbness, tears, and reflection both poignant and comical: "These spectators watched as I visualized my death, with probable accuracy, for the first time. And the picture was so banal. . . . I'd never play Rummikub with Bill Clinton or have my own self-titled sitcom and theme song? My son wouldn't know his mother? I'd just be that unphotogenic woman pawing at him in all those pictures" (32). Ironic self-deprecation is juxtaposed here with fantasies of thwarted fame and maternal loss, strategies that produce a tragicomic effect. However, since we know that Norton survives to write this book, readers can downplay the tragedy of her diagnosis and laugh at her self-representation. One of Norton's most salient themes is the grueling side effects of chemotherapy, which she recounts via the strategy of comic excess. Although nausea is the most immediate aftermath of chemo for many cancer patients, an effective medication allows Norton to bypass this symptom and concentrate instead on her stinky urine, about which she waxes poetic.

> I took a tiny antinausea pill and within minutes, miraculously, simply felt hungover. I lay down, turned out the lights, and slept dreamlessly until morning. Then I got up and peed the most noxious-smelling urine imaginable. It wasn't even yellow, but grayish-brown, like water emptied from a steam cleaner. . . . Even though I drank till my belly felt stretched beyond capacity, the smell of my urine was so potent it made my eyes water. It slowly evolved into a meaty, rotten odor, slightly sweet and bloody smelling. (43)

Norton's graphic imagery and excessive bodily revelation produce in readers the horrified "ugh" that she no doubt anticipates as a writer adopting the style of stand-up comedians who use the comic grotesque to evoke laughter.[3]

Equally reliant on the comic grotesque is Norton's rendering of chemo-induced hair loss. "A hairless body has its appeal," she admits disarmingly, "but losing eyelashes and eyebrows just looks creepy" (44). An experience in the shower shortly after her second treatment robs Norton of the illusion that unlike other chemo patients, she will retain her hair. After noticing "an awful lot of hair on my bar of soap, and on my shoulders, and between my toes," she combs her hair only to find it "clogged full with each stroke. My scalp tingled. It was strangely satisfying. My hair felt so thin, my skull so close, but when I looked in the mirror I could hardly see the difference" (45). The difference emerges a few days later, however, during a trip to Target with a friend.

> There, in front of the Hello Kitty party invitations, I reached to scratch over my ear and all the hair, clear to my temple, peeled off, like a piece of Velcro. It even made that ripping Velcro sound.

> Rebecca stared in amazement, and then I peeled off the other one. We stood in the stationery and office supply section holding the two stiff patches and laughed until our cheeks ached. (46)

The use of simile drives Norton's chemo humor—urine smelling like a steam cleaner's filthy water, hair peeling off like Velcro—along with her ironic references to American consumer culture, here represented by Target and Hello Kitty. Although she admits to feeling traumatized when her friend cuts what little hair remains, Norton deflects her pain through strategic self-deprecation—"this baldness made me officially the least desirable woman alive"—and through sexualized humor: "She shaved off what was left of my ego and Thibault's id while I held Lucas on my lap" (47). Maternity as well as laughter sustains Norton, as her infant son chortles while his mother's hair falls, "lunging for the little disposable razor to shave my head himself" (47). Rebellious humor thus allows the narrator to highlight poignant domestic moments without evoking reader pity.

Her response to medicalization, an ambivalent blend of resistance and compliance, provides Norton with another humorous subject. The daughter of a urologist, she is predisposed to trust the judgment of her consulting physicians, yet their frantic pace and dubious bedside manners sometimes give her pause. The surgeon scheduled to perform Norton's mastectomy, for example, receives this blunt assessment.

> She did the training, passed the exams, got the degrees, and had the authority to pump me full of toxins and chop off my breasts. I had no choice but to lie still and trust she wasn't too distracted by her house's termite problem to confuse me with the lobotomy patient at 9:30. (117)

Notwithstanding her apparent acquiescence, Norton brings in her father to interrogate Dr. Ree about the possibility of a nonsurgical approach: "'Have you considered that?' His tone grew more combative. Dr. Ree's voice stayed controlled, but her clenched fists betrayed her defensiveness. 'Some reports suggest higher locoregional failure rates—'" When Dr. Norton interrupts Dr. Ree to protest that he doesn't "give a damn about local control" but is concerned only about his daughter's survival, Norton acknowledges her mistake in initiating this conversation and

watches in horror as her father risks alienating the surgeon—an alienation avoided by Dr. Norton's sudden tears of worry for his daughter and
Dr. Ree's sympathetic response (116–17). num of as genial
coping
    Norton also uses self-deprecating humor to mock the denial she
engages as a stage-three breast-cancer patient. She twice postpones her
scheduled mastectomy in the wild hope that conversations with patholo-
gists would prove she had actually never had cancer (those slides "could
have said lupus or shingles or anything") or that online research would
offer some alternative. Realizing retrospectively that her resistance marks
a terrified delusion, Norton reveals her gradual acceptance of mastectomy. In one instance of strategic self-deprecation, the narrator praises
the long-suffering Dr. Ree: "Not once did she scream, 'You moron with
your Internet medical degree! Stop questioning me!' She just nodded her
head when I canceled my surgery and thought to herself, 'You poor, stupid dolt.' Then she quietly rescheduled it when I called her back" (125–
26). In other passages Norton praises her surgeon's wizardry in comic
terms, three days after surgery, for example, when the patient insists on
viewing her post-mastectomy scar.

> I led her into the little bathroom. She unswaddled my rib cage
> slowly. Finally, there it was. On the left side sat my smashed flat,
> deflated boob, and on the right side, nothing, just a thin line of
> steri-strip tape over the actual incision. Flat as a wall. There were
> no black stitches, no gruesome scar. . . . "You are a freaking magi-
> cian! I so should have gone to medical school." I looked at it from
> every angle. (140)

Agency rests here with the irrepressible Norton, who delights in her surgeon's feat, accepts her new body, and laments not her absent breast but
her lack of a medical degree.
    Another focus for Norton's satiric humor is her frustration with
mainstream survivor discourse. One source of irritation is the theatrics
of strange women she encounters in breast cancer support groups or
public spaces, "cancer survivors who expected me to feel some sort of
camaraderie."

> They would clasp my hands tightly and demand that I curse this
> disease, this awful scourge. I tried, but couldn't do it with any

heart. . . . But it seemed so disrespectful to tell another cancer patient, "Let go of my hands, you kook!" that I almost always acqui-
esced and lazily stamped my feet and said sternly "Bad cancer!" I
felt like an idiot every time, and every time vowed to never do it
again. Then some other random bald person would approach me
at the grocery store or car wash and rope me into this lame ritual
all over again. (58)

In this passage Norton nails the dilemma of patients eager to resist cancer culture's oppressive cheerfulness yet caught up in its endless self-
replication. Strategic self-deprecation takes the edge off her otherwise
trenchant critique of New Age approaches to healing and empowerment.

Norton also locks rhetorical horns with one of survivor discourse's
most famous purveyors, Lance Armstrong, whose inspirational cancer
memoir she receives as a gift from countless friends but with whom she
feels no affinity.

Lance Armstrong and I are close to exact opposites, both physically and mentally. . . . If surviving this particularly deadly form of
breast cancer required any of the Lance-like traits, such as willingness to physically exert myself, I was as good as dead. What I really
needed to save me from utter despondency was to see somebody
who's never taken life by the horns, for no better reason than complacency, remain true to himself and still beat cancer, someone
like every character ever played by Bill Murray. (book jacket)

This witty put-down of the compulsively driven Armstrong, victorious
over multiple cancers and the Tour de France, in favor of the laconic
losers played by Murray pivots on comic incongruity and the ironic de-
flation of the culturally sanctioned approach to beating cancer through
willpower.[4] A recurring figure in Norton's text, Armstrong serves mostly
as a whipping boy, as she determines to "poke a stick in Lance's spoke" for
upholding unrealistic standards of cancer patient behavior.

Lance Armstrong has excessive drive and talent. His motivation
and discipline grow like crab grass and dandelions. I just don't
have it like that. Every day of my chemo that I ate a Krispy Kreme
doughnut or took a nap instead of doing yoga I cursed Lance

> Armstrong and his toned abs, tiny butt, and three kinds of cancer. "F you, Lance Armstrong," I muttered as I sucked down my Dr. Pepper. "You can park your bike right here and kiss my ass." (133)

Saucy defiance and colloquial vulgarity merge in this passage, as laughing readers relish Norton's exaggerated representation. Near the end of her memoir, however, Norton rehabilitates Armstrong as a celebrity to commend—not because of his triumph over cancer or championship cycling but because of his angry claim that the players on the French 2006 FIFA World Cup Team all "tested positive . . . for being assholes" (92, 209). Because Armstrong mouthed off in public, Norton concludes, "he was officially my hero" (209). Here she comically redefines heroism as backtalk.

Norton's memoir concludes by recounting two family celebrations: a "Meredith Kills Cancer Dead" party to celebrate her "victory" (a term she employs ironically), held unfortunately on the very evening her oncologist determines that she needs another aggressive round of chemo; and her son's fourth birthday party, held on the third anniversary of her breast cancer diagnosis (157). Norton refuses to bring closure to her narrative—"Nothing else has happened, but it will. As my father says, 'None of us gets out of here alive'"—yet she celebrates her temporary reprieve, since "statistics suggested I wouldn't live to see my son turn four" (210–11). While she resists being labeled a survivor, she acknowledges wryly having lived through much, from the racist indignity of being repeatedly mistaken for a prostitute in Paris to a realization that despite the promises made by mainstream cancer culture, her illness had made her no wiser. Her memoir foregrounds not false cheerfulness but a wry wit and a bemused hope that she might live long enough to pursue a PhD and see her son grow up.

Comic Relief in *Cancer Made Me a Shallower Person*

A cartoonist by profession, Miriam Engelberg wrote for several years in the mid-1990s a widely circulated comic series, *Planet 501c3*, designed to inform and encourage employees of U.S. nonprofit organizations. When diagnosed with breast cancer, she understandably turned to comics as a mode of self-examination.

> We all have issues that follow us through life, no matter how much therapy we've had. The big one for me is about feeling different and alone—isolated in a state of Miriam-ness that no one else experiences. That's what drew me to read autobiographical comics, and that's why I hope my comics can be of comfort to other readers who might be struggling with issues similar to mine. (xiii)

Although she describes her purpose as communal and therapeutic, her tone in *Cancer Made Me a Shallower Person* remains light and often self-mocking. Acknowledging in her introduction that perhaps "someday I'll have something profound to say" about cancer and suffering, at the initial moment of writing she privileges distraction over profundity: "right now I have to go—it's time to watch *Celebrity Poker*" (xiii). Strategic self-deprecation is evident in her positioning of the narrative *I* as addicted to popular culture and deficient in seriousness of purpose.

As Hillary Chute notes in *Graphic Women*, "some of the most riveting feminist cultural production is in the form of accessible yet edgy graphic narratives"—a postmillennial genre that offers a new aesthetics of gendered self-representation (2). As one salient example of this type of cultural production, Engelberg's narrative constitutes what Chute characterizes as a "cross-discursive form," a capacious medium in which "words and images entwine, but never synthesize" (6, 9). Through the device of frames, or "boxes of time," the graphic artist presents a visual/verbal text "threaded with absence, with the rich white spaces of what is called the gutter" and yet filled as well with the "subjective mark" of the maker's drawings and handwriting (Chute, 10). The result is a richly textured narrative that constitutes "an expanded idiom of witness"—a method of testimony, Chute concludes, that "sets a visual language in motion with and against the verbal in order to embody individual and collective experience, to put contingent selves and histories into form" (3).

To understand why and how graphic narratives can effectively represent not only the traumatic but also the irreverent aspects of the cancer experience, it is useful to consider the analysis of medical humanities scholar Martha Stoddard Holmes, who notes that the pop-culture genre of *comix,* used as a term to designate humorous sequential art, has links both to mainstream American domesticity, in that traditional U.S. families have for generations shared and enjoyed the Sunday funnies, and to radical underground works of political satire from the 1960s and beyond. "What attributes of this medium lend it so well to telling cancer stories?" she asks, pointing out that whereas the "connection between comics and humor is not hard wired, it is a default expectation because of the divergent terms"—the incongruity, that is, between having *fun* and having *cancer*. Yet many cancer patients engage humor not for therapy but because their bodily changes and medicalization inevitably produce moments worthy of laughter. According to Stoddard Holmes, autobiographical breast cancer comics typically feature four distinguishing characteristics: (1) they "figure the self iconically" rather than realistically, a strategy that allows the ill subject to reshape her identity as the disease progresses and invites reader identification with the patient's cartoon face and shape-shifting capacity; (2) they "render time as space" by offering a narrative that is at once visual and verbal, one in which past and future are visible even as the present provides stress or release; (3) they create a "materiality of language" that erases the distinctions among speech, fantasy, and imagination and that may be especially apt for representing the disorienting effects of "chemo brain"; and (4) they both *use* closure, by concluding each cartoon sequence with a witty denouement, and *refuse* closure, by ending the final cartoon frame inconclusively to signify the uncertainties of living with/beyond cancer. In this regard, cancer comics "elide the cure narrative" that dominates more conventional forms of cancer memoirs (Stoddard Holmes).[5]

Cancer Made Me a Shallower Person presents a woman who survives mastectomy and chemotherapy only to learn that her cancer has metastasized to her bones and brain. Readers who look online can learn that Engelberg died in 2006, shortly after her book was published. Her cancer narrative displays many of the features discussed by Stoddard Holmes, as is evident from an analysis of three representative cartoons. The first, an eighteen-frame sequence positioned early in the book and entitled *Diagnosis,* transforms the conventional "why me?" mantra into an ironic "what did I do to cause this?" meditation. *Diagnosis* juggles playful self-deprecation and implicit cultural critique. "Before getting my biopsy results everyone was very encouraging," explains the iconic Miriam, a black-and-white line-drawn Everywoman with shoulder-length curly hair, wire-rimmed glasses, and an indeterminate age. The word balloons that emerge from the mouths of eight well-meaning but clueless friends recount such banal anecdotes as "my mom and my sister both had calcification, and it wasn't cancer!"; "I had the same thing and it was benign, it's no big deal"; and "my cat had a lump, but . . ." (np). Miriam's narrative, rendered in a word stream at the top of each square frame, acknowledges her increasing irritation at such comments. Her downturned mouth and the thought bubble that appears in frame two raise the cartoon's blame-the-victim motif: "Are they saying I'm being overly dramatic? Am I worrying over nothing?" When the physician's phone call comes with the news that it is indeed breast cancer, Miriam has two simultaneous reactions: "Oh my God! I can't believe it. This is horrible!" (words she says to her doctor) and "Ha! *Now* they'll take me seriously!" (her fantasy as she imagines confrontations with disbelieving friends). Readers can identify with Miriam's cartoon face and her incongruous responses to the bad news, as Engelberg's effective blend of words and images allows representations of the "real" and the imaginary to coexist.

Having redeemed herself by contracting cancer, Miriam narrates her unsuccessful struggle "to restrain my tell-all tendencies"—in frame six she responds to a casual acquaintance's "Hi! How are you?" by sobbing "I have breast cancer!"—and to determine which of her behaviors might have caused her disease. Caricature abounds, as Miriam envisions the judgment of her health-conscious parents ("We walk 3 miles a day, do tai chi and take megavitamins," brags the wide-eyed, smiling maternal figure), parents who "for years . . . have been mailing me articles," from recipes for health to information about "fat linked to cancer" (np). Parody and self-deprecation abound as Miriam proceeds relentlessly past possible environmental causes and toward self-blame. "I caused this by eating too much cheese. . . . All their health stuff was right after all. I never should have relaxed and enjoyed life," she laments in one thought bubble, a numb expression on her face, hands lifted in disbelief (np). Grocery shopping in subsequent frames, she rejects toxic fish, hormone-filled meats, dairy products, and sugar, and ends up buying simply a bottle of water, only to wonder, "Uh oh, did I read that bottled water can have high levels of arsenic?" With characteristic hyperbole, Miriam (rendered in profile, grim and determined, as she pushes her cart past all temptations) concludes that "the only safe solution is to stop eating!" (np).

In the final four frames, reassured by friends that she is not to blame for her cancer, Miriam narrates her perverse discovery of new ways to affirm her guilt. To the concerned companion who reminds her, over tea, that "the Bay Area has one of the highest breast cancer rates in the world," the cartoon Miriam replies, "You're right. I never should have moved here. It's all my fault!!" Thus she comically pretends to reject environmental causes in favor of lifestyle. To her cancer support group she confesses, "I think I caused this by eating too much cheese," only to be teased by comrades who acknowledge feeling guilty for repressing anger, taking birth control pills, or painting with oils. The final frame's discourse raises matters ontological—"It's hard not to keep wondering about the cause. But would it really help to know?" This frame consists of line drawings of a seated Miriam gazing up at a standing physician of ambiguous status and gender, recognizable by a stethoscope around his/her neck. Returning to ironic self-blame, Engelberg represents the verdict in a word balloon emerging from the doctor's mouth: "This DNA test reveals conclusively that a cheese-induced gene mutation caused your cancer. In layman's terms, it was all your fault" (np). Miriam's presentation of her grateful response parodies the hierarchical conventions of the doctor-patient dynamic and reinforces Engelberg's theme—the absurdity yet the cultural ubiquity of blaming cancer patients for contracting their disease: "Thanks for telling me. Now I'll be able to sink into a really deep depression" (np). This cartoon sequence illustrates the comic strategy of "amplification through simplification," in Scott McCloud's words, the presentation of a dominant idea through concrete detail and iconic abstraction to effect a "stripped down intensity" that promotes reader identification through laughter (30).

Midway through the book Engelberg takes on tyrannical cheerfulness in *Something Unpleasant and You,* which satirizes the ubiquitous educational booklets that represent chemotherapy as a benign process that will leave a compliant breast cancer patient feeling energetic and healed. In this twelve-frame sequence readers see the figure of Miriam change from curly-haired and smiling to bald and weeping; we experience time rendered as space, since both the hairless Miriam of "now" and the full-haired Miriam of "then" coincide in this sequence; and we recognize linguistic materiality in the juxtaposed representations of Miriam's world versus booklet world. The cover art invites particular comic scrutiny: a booklet entitled *Chemotherapy and You,* for example, rendered in frame two, features a calm ocean, a palm tree, and a cavorting dolphin on its cover, to which the iconic Miriam responds in frame three's word balloon, "I was dreading chemo, but now that I can associate it with this lovely beach scene I'm looking forward to it!" In frame four Engelberg critiques another booklet cover, *Breast Cancer Surgery . . . and You!* with

SOMETHING UNPLEASANT AND YOU

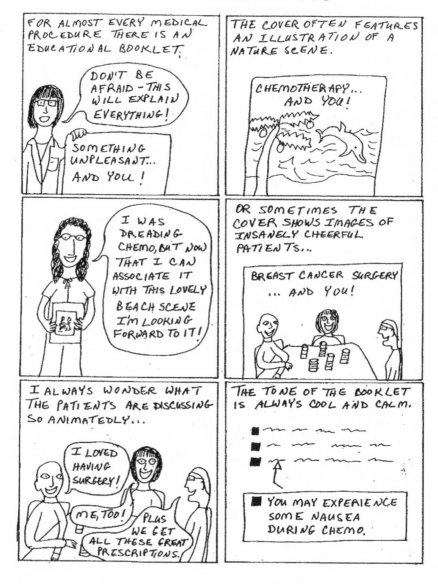

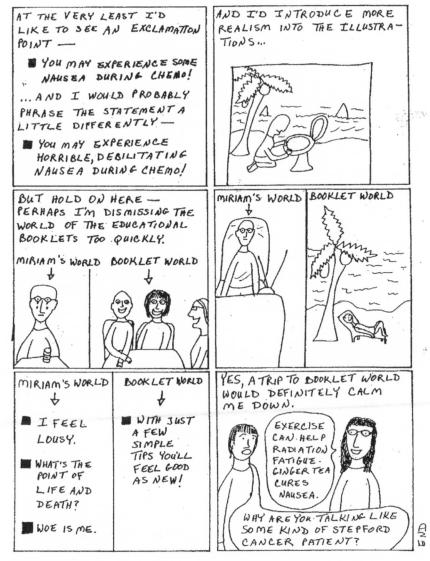

Miriam Engelberg, "Something Unpleasant and You,"
pp. 40–41. From *Cancer Made Me a Shallower Person: A Memoir in Comics*, c. 2006. Reprinted by permission of HarperCollins Publishers.

three smiling women—one wigged, another scarved, a third bald—discussing how much they enjoyed their surgeries. "Plus we get all these great prescriptions," the woman wearing the scarf intones, revealing another satiric subject for cancer memoirists, their debilitating drugs. "The tone of the booklet is always cool and calm," Miriam's pseudo-objective narration continues, as frame six advises the patient reading the booklet that "you may experience some nausea during chemo" (np).

Dissatisfied with this optimistic information, the iconic Miriam rewrites the booklet copy in frame seven—"You may experience horrible, debilitating nausea during chemo!"—and in frame eight depicts a bald woman about to vomit into a toilet on a shark-infested beach. In frames nine and ten Engelberg uses a split-frame device to differentiate her solitary grief from the forced cheerfulness of such booklets and to distinguish Miriam's grim hospital room from the booklet's idealized seaside setting. The language Engelberg employs here is terse and pessimistic, albeit exaggeratedly so: "I feel lousy," Miriam exclaims, "What's the point of life and death?" She also resorts to the cliché "Woe is me." The contrasting language of booklet world is stereotypical, upbeat, and infantilizing: "With just a few simple tips, you'll feel good as new" (np). Despite her doubts, the narrative Miriam admits sardonically in the final frame, "a trip to booklet world would definitely calm me down"—though at the price of becoming a "Stepford cancer patient" (np). As McCloud notes, "comic panels fracture both time and space," and in this sequence Engelberg engages temporal and spatial imagery to launch an uproarious journey through the unrealistic world of breast cancer booklets.

Themes of recurrence and metastasis rarely appear in humorous breast cancer memoirs, since laughter is positioned culturally as a tool of the not-dying, and death is nothing to laugh about. For Engelberg, however, a recurrence in the form of bone and brain metastases provides opportunity for gallows humor. In *A Potpourri of Scans* the iconic Miriam reveals the distressing news of her dual "mets" but also jokes about the appalling noises of MRI machines, the confusing directions for putting on a "3-armed gown," and the naive encouragement of friends. In this eighteen-frame cartoon near the end of the memoir Engelberg takes the trope of self-division to gruesome heights.[6] Miriam confides in frame one that "there is a divide in the breast cancer community" and illustrates that claim with a circle divided by a lightning-bolt line, one side labeled "primary diagnosis only" (to which her response is "I'm OK—really"), the other side labeled "gone metastatic" (to which she responds "damn!"). Despite attempts by the oncologist to reassure Miriam that a cancerous lymph node signifies local recurrence, a subsequent CAT scan reveals bone metastasis. The scan itself, however, is humorously rendered in frames four through seven, as Miriam struggles to don impossible garments required for the procedure, tries in vain to heed the warning printed on the machine—"laser beam, do not stare into aperture!"—and speculates that the laser beam "improved my eyesight" (np). A follow-up MRI, depicted in frames nine through eleven, presents a prone Miriam entering yet another alienating machine, grim in contrast to the smiling technician at her side. Through sound bubbles Engelberg represents the machine's disconcerting noises—"BOOM-A BOOM-A-BOOM-A-BOOM-A," "CLACK CLACK CLACK," "PLINK PLINK"—which lead Miriam to "picture the Monty Python team out in the control room making sound effects" (np).

The last six frames, which reveal the presence of brain metastasis, unsettle reader-viewers as Engelberg uses strategies of comic disruption to shift her narrative trajectory from restitution to autothanatography. These drawings present an open-mouthed figure responding with horror to her oncologist's phone call—"In my brain? Oh my God!"—as her wide-eyed husband cries "Oh no!" The narrowing world that the iconic Miriam inhabits is once again represented through a circular drawing; here the "gone metastatic" half of the earlier circle is further subdivided into a fragment that reads, "Anyone in there?" This lonely query reflects the isolation Miriam experiences at the news of her brain metastasis, as her odds of survival diminish. Grim irony prevails as the cartoonist represents her alter ego rejecting inspirational messages and confronting optimistic friends with a placard that reads, "Lance Armstrong had a different form of cancer!" Like Norton, Engelberg resists Armstrong as cancer's fetishized spokesperson and claims agency by distinguishing her experience from his. Although denial can provide only temporary solace, she returns to it in the final frame, as the iconic Miriam tries to convince herself that if Monty Python was indeed operating the MRI machine, "maybe I didn't *really* have brain mets." Such allusions to popular culture reinforce Engelberg's introductory claim that she would be not the "heroic type of cancer patient portrayed in so many television shows and movies" but one who "looked for pop culture distraction" (xii). In choosing transgressive humor over tragic angst as a strategy for representing metastatic cancer, the cartoonist confronts death with comic equanimity yet refuses to conceal her fear and grief.

Blogging and Kvetching in *The Adventures of Cancer Bitch*

If breast cancer often begins with a "whiff of criminality," as S. L. Wisenberg alleges in a blog entitled "Cells Gone Wild," so does her 2009 memoir *The Adventures of Cancer Bitch,* which boasts cancer as subversive muse and uses strategic narcissism as narrative strategy (2). Having posted nearly five hundred blogs between 2007 and 2010 on CancerBitchblogspot.com, this defiant memoirist invites readers into a landscape demarcated by spatial word coinages: Fancy Hospital, home of Fancy Surgeon, toward whom she feels ambivalent; Plain Hospital, where a Much Recommended Surgeon practices; Chemolandia, where Wisenberg wows her sister infusion patients with a tattooed bald head; and Cancer Bitch World Headquarters, where she seduces readers by kvetching about the sentimentality of mainstream breast cancer culture and the perils of teaching one-breasted. In a retrospective essay about her illness blogs, Wisenberg playfully acknowledges that contracting breast cancer fed her ego: "There is a delight? Can I say that? That I'm center stage? That something dramatic has happened. . . . That's what it is. That's what I don't want to tell anybody. That I'm important because the killer has lodged in me" ("Bitching and Blogging," 20). That ego is fragile at best, however, and quite possibly a performative ruse; in her subsequent memoir Wisenberg acknowledges fear, depression, and bodily insecurity, all of which she deflects through wit. A wily blend of self-aggrandizement and self-deflation thus fuels her comic voice.

Wisenberg engages a more anti-pink discourse in her memoir than does either Norton or Engelberg, in part because she writes from a more explicitly feminist standpoint. As an advocate of Breast Cancer Action (BCA) and its environmentally focused critiques of corporate cancer culture, Wisenberg challenges tight pink T-shirts that sexualize the disease and multinational corporations that "hop on the Pink bandwagon" by selling "Pink Ribbon Cupcakes and Support the Cause Brownies" (*Adventures,* 5). She uses irony to highlight the absurdity of buying pink M&M's ("That's all I eat. If I eat enough of them my cancer will go away") or attending Avon Walks to promote breast cancer awareness ("Do I get a free Avon makeover before setting out: all those cameras, you see; I must look my best?") (5). Instead of consumerism and walkathons, she recommends joining Code Pink, a feminist antiwar group, or reading Samantha King's treatise *Pink Ribbons, Inc.: Breast Cancer and the Politics of Philanthropy*, which posits that the "Komen Foundation and its corporate sponsors continue to pump money into a research and education agenda that is . . . actually doing more harm than good" (6). Wisenberg's pink-bashing continues throughout the blog-turned-memoir, as she ridicules Fancy Hospital for giving away a "free (!) pink emery board" at the front desk of its Cancer Floor: "What is the purpose of a pink emery board? To remind you to have a mammogram when you're sawing down your nails? In general the pink ribbon thing is supposed to make you Feel Feminine even though you've lost the outward manifestation of what men think of as feminine in this country. Thank you, Hugh Hefner" (35). Yet she acknowledges that while she prefers BCA's anticorporatism to market-driven philanthropy, her anger at the "Pink Ribbon people" might be misplaced, since even the Komen Foundation began in grief and was thus once "pure" (39).[7]

Like other feminist autobiographers, Wisenberg embraces baldness and one-breastedness as strategies for evading the pressures of hegemonic femininity. Having refused to fill a prescription for a "cranial prosthesis" (aka wig), she recounts sporting a Mohawk once her hair loss begins, tattooing her bald head with leaf-shaped henna swirls and peace signs, using her scalp as an antiwar billboard to proclaim "US Out of Iraq," and presenting herself proudly to sister bloggers as "just another bald-headed girl for peace" (*Adventures*, 74). She mocks the trauma of becoming "Un-Mohawked" when her remaining tufts of hair fall out midway through chemo and endorses "The Bad Girls of Breast Cancer" who wear black T-shirts with an X over the missing breast rather than pink ones labeled "Breast Buddies" or "Under Reconstruction," captions she deems "suitable only for Hooters customers" (76, 37). She parodies mainstream culture's sexualization of breasts by hosting a Farewell to My Left Breast Party the night before her mastectomy that features frothy breasted figures on its dessert menu: cream puffs with candy nipples, giant Hershey kisses, scoops of peach ice cream topped with cherries. Although she decides against breast reconstruction, she admits struggling over this decision: "I have to admit that I've been feeling lazy for not replacing my breast. Maybe feeling lazy and slatternly for going around braless and one-breastless. O gosh, lost a breast and didn't even sew one back on. As if it were a button fallen off a coat" (137). In these wry passages the memoirist defies gender norms, destigmatizes one-breastedness, and ridicules the cultural obsession with breasts.

In her boldest defiance of post-mastectomy etiquette, Wisenberg employs ribald humor to recount her pubic hair loss due to chemotherapy. This taboo confession opens with a description of the first hairs she found in her bathtub, which "looked like a swarm of ants," and culminates with an explicit account of her bald pubis and visible labia (*Adventures*, 73). In a blog entitled "The Million Dollar Brazilian" she riffs on the increasingly popular grooming practice among young U.S. women of having their pubic hair waxed. "Why?" she wonders, only to report that research reveals "men want women to be bare because they want their sex partners to look like porn stars" (102). Unsurprisingly, she embraces neither the J. Sisters Salon in New York, cited in *Marie Claire* magazine as a prime site, nor the porn aesthetic of pubis-waxing.

> Cancer Bitch has never waxed anything, including floors and furniture, though in her youth she bleached her mustache and arm hairs. Now she doesn't have to because Adriamycin and Taxol have left her hair-depleted. She has two half-eyebrows, just a little hair left on her shins, and a threadbare little nest above her crotch. How can I say this delicately? There's a slit underneath the nest. It reminds her of the profile of a crocodile. (*Adventures*, 102–3)

Revealing the comic details of her shorn pubis, Wisenberg admits to worry over whether the administration of Fancy University, where she teaches but lacks tenure, will fire her for pornographic commentary. Ultimately she reassures herself that academic freedom will protect her and that "after all, this is why the second wave of feminists fought, so that in the early 21st century, a Cancer Bitch could write about her loss of pubic hair with impunity" (*Adventures*, 103).

A prominent narrative strategy in *The Adventures of Cancer Bitch* is the cross-referencing of feminist writers and artists who have challenged the breast cancer marketplace. Although Wisenberg mentions celebrities with breast cancer such as Sheryl Crow and Gilda Radner, her praise is reserved for feminist critics of cancer culture, most notably Barbara Ehrenreich, Deena Metzger, Matuschka, and Miriam Engelberg. Ehrenreich's oft-cited essay "Welcome to Cancerland," published in *Harper's* in 2001, exposed what Wisenberg characterizes as "too much treacle out there about breast cancer—positive attitudes, what my cancer taught me" (*Adventures*, 23). Metzger's exuberant photograph of her one-breasted tattooed chest, taken in 1976 by Hella Hammid, attracts Wisenberg through its iconic status in feminist breast cancer history, although she refuses to tattoo her own chest because it "would hurt too much" (28). Matuschka's *Beauty Out of Damage,* which appeared on the cover of the *New York Times* magazine in 1993, captures Wisenberg's attention for its brave self-portraiture, "a woman taking a picture of her own scarred self after her breast was cut away" (139). And Engelberg's *Cancer Made Me a Shallower Person* appeals to Wisenberg because the cartoonist stares at death with humor: "There is always the void. Let's laugh to cover it up" (33).

In contrast to her praise of feminist pioneers, Wisenberg ridicules women she considers breast cancer's public glamour girls: Cancer Vixen (the New Yorker cartoonist and cancer memoirist Marisa Acocella Marchetto, although she is never named); the authors of the Skinny Bitch vegan cookbook (also unnamed), for whom thinness is a major goal; anyone who values the trappings of femininity over health.

> I'm not going to be like those superficial fucking girls who live for their cleavage, who won't take tamoxifen because they might gain weight, and the reason they can't gain weight is because their appearance is more important than their survival. I don't want to be like Cancer Vixen who just thinks about shoes and hair. I want to be like Miriam Engelberg but she died. I'm crying. I'm crying for her because the one I want to be like died. (*Adventures,* 45)

Grief at Engelberg's death blends here with strategic narcissism as Wisenberg both laments and laughs at her own mortality.

Wisenberg's Jewish identity is as central to her narrative as is her feminist politics. As she confronts mastectomy and chemotherapy, she studies the Torah, attends Passover seders, commemorates Yom Kippur, and reads texts of Jewish mysticism. Reflections on Judaism provide much of her serious subject matter, in particular the shame that many Jews associate with bald heads because of forcible shavings of the heads of Jewish women and men by the Nazis during the Holocaust. In addition, her status as an Ashkenazi Jew leads Wisenberg to be tested for BRCA1 and BRCA2 mutations, and the topic of genetic predisposition toward breast and ovarian cancers occupies her even after her test results come back negative. Her often sober meditations on Judaism and the Holocaust also reveal subversive humor.

> For some American Jews, the Holocaust is our holy of holies. Auschwitz is our version of the crucifixion, and we approach it, the idea of it, with horrified awe. . . . The Holocaust is my automatic reference point to many things—if it's really cold outside I think about morning roll calls in dark dead winter in Poland in the death camps. . . . I wrote a book called *Holocaust Girls,* about people (like myself) who identify with the Holocaust too much.
>
> That's why the term is a household word now.
>
> (You mean it's not?) (*Adventures,* 9)

In this passage Wisenberg uses her cultural identification with the Holocaust as a narrative tool for meditating on the horrors of genocide but also for lamenting her previous book's lack of a sufficiently large academic audience.

Unlike Norton and Engelberg, who never analyze their own comic strategies, Wisenberg reflects on the role of laughter in her narrative confrontation with breast cancer. While she is initially drawn to nervous laughter as a coping mechanism, she later rejects it as evasive.

> I hate nervous laughter. It seems so fake. It seems to be covering up. It seems to be negating what you're saying. I don't want to be a nervous laugher. I remember talking to someone a few years ago about her mastectomy and she was all barky nervous laughter. It put me off. But I am doing it. I'm getting a part of my body cut off, ha-ha. If the cancer has spread I could die, ha-ha. (*Adventures,* 31–32)

Wisenberg does acknowledges the power of catalytic laughter as a form of release—for example, she enjoys making audiences laugh aloud when she reads from her memoir: "It's easy to make a happy, willing crowd laugh. They want to laugh. They need it, to let off steam, from their waiting, their wanting. The nervousness of all being together, chairs set up in rows, side by side. All the raggedy breathing. . . . We are animals that need to make noise" (*Adventures,* 32). Here she posits what Andrew Stott identifies as the relief theory of laughter, which pivots on "a struggle of incongruous selfhood" in defiance of both cultural and unconscious taboos (131). In his work on comic theory Stott reminds readers that Freud viewed laughter as a means of alleviating inhibitions: "Laughing is the audible signal of energy required for cathexis," which can in turn restore

mental equilibrium (131). Wisenberg concurs, and she uses humor strategically in her narrative to evoke reader connection and relief: "Enough
of memoirs about trauma and sorrow and addiction" (*Adventures,* 23).

In her retrospective essay "Bitching and Blogging Through Breast
Cancer" Wisenberg reflects on her lifelong preoccupation with suffering,
her chronic depression, and her reasons for writing the blogs that became her memoir. If in a journal "you strip yourself down as close to the
bone as possible," in a blog you "can look both inward and outward, because it's theoretically available to every single person on the planet who's
online" (21). Her postings served as "a journal with benefits," since she
could write not only to complain about her post-mastectomy drainage
tubes or ponder mortality but also to amuse herself and others: "And—I
know how this sounds—I wrote about the fun I had with cancer" (21).
For Wisenberg, blogs replaced therapy: "I felt listened to even on days
when friends, as well as strangers such as Colon Cancer Cowgirl and The
Fifty-foot Woman, didn't give feedback in the comments section" (21).
Kvetching about breast cancer thus provided laughs and a lifeline.

The Cultural Capital of Transgressive Laughter

Why laugh about breast cancer? One answer can be found in the medical
websites and journals that surface when one investigates cancer, laughter,
and humor. A 2006 article by Mary Payne Bennett and Cecile Lengacher,
"Humor and Laughter May Influence Health: Complementary Therapies
and Humor in a Clinical Population," featured at a website supported
by the National Institutes of Health, notes that in a survey of 105 breast
cancer patient-respondents in Florida, 21 percent used laughter as a
"complementary and alternative medicine," while in a smaller study 50
percent of patients found the use of medical humor helpful during treatment (pubmedcentral.nih.gov). Such studies represent the most recent
manifestation of a long history of medical endorsement of the healing
power of laughter, beginning with Hippocrates, the "laughing philosopher" of ancient Greece who viewed laughter as an antidote to disease
(Stott, 131). Comedy cures, as one often-visited cancer humor website
proclaims, however exaggeratedly.[8] Increasingly in postmillennial medical culture, humor therapy, web-based jokes and games, comic memoirs,
and laughter-inducing activities are being prescribed to help breast cancer patients cope, heal, and even face death with defiance or equanimity.

While Norton, Engelberg, and Wisenberg are among the best-known published authors of comic memoirs, the blogosphere abounds with feminist breast cancer humor. For example, an October 30, 2008, posting on assertivepatient.com by Jeanne Sather, "Introducing Breast Cancer Joe," explains why she is launching a new product for the men of America.

> In 2006, in October, of course, Mattel introduced Breast Cancer Barbie. I bought one to add to my Wall of Shame, and she's been there ever since, raising awareness in a different way from what Mattel intended. . . . I thought at the time that if I did a gender-reversal people might better be able to see how stupid this Barbie doll is, and how offensive it is to a woman like me. . . . Because men do get breast cancer. No one thinks about that when they open clinics to treat breast cancer where the only backless gowns available to patients—male and female—are pink. (Sather)

Using pink-bashing to take on the toy industry and the breast cancer marketplace, Sather provides photographs of Mattel's Barbie (both pointed breasts intact) and her own stiff-torsoed Joe, clad in a rose-colored helmet and looking stoic. The box caption that accompanies her product reveals that Joe "comes with the following accessories: pink helmet, boots, backless pink camouflage hospital gown, pink teddy bear, military issue weapon, repainted pink, pink hand grenade, and pink ribbon tattoo" (Sather). If G.I. Joe could survive Vietnam, surely Breast Cancer Joe can handle chemotherapy.

Like Ehrenreich, who underwent treatment for breast cancer in 2001 and became offended by the endless array of ultrafeminine and infantilizing products she encountered, Sather uses her authority as a breast cancer patient to object to crass marketing ploys.

> As a woman living with breast cancer (and minus one breast) who is forced to run a gauntlet of pink products every October, my question is this: What does this beauty queen, fairy princess DOLL in a pink formal gown say about me and my experience with breast cancer?
> And the answer is: Nothing. Nothing.
> This doll does not offer me hope.

> This doll certainly does not offer a positive image of a strong woman living with cancer.
>
> And the doll is not even a fund-raising effort that I can support. (Sather)

The blogger cheekily suggests revisions to Breast Cancer Barbie should Mattel truly want to fulfill its stated goal of inspiring women with this disease: "If Barbie were to represent us, she should be bald, and come with an assortment of wigs and headscarves—the fashionistas at Mattel who created the 'sparkly tulle stole that evokes the iconic pink ribbon' missed that one. . . . Breast Cancer Barbie would also need that essential chemo accessory: a small pink toilet in which to upchuck when nausea strikes" (Sather).

Transgressive breast cancer humor has also pervaded YouTube, primarily through performance art by comedians who bare their souls and chests for laughs. Queer performance artist and writer Tania Katan, for example, includes on her website links to a YouTube segment in which she lectures shirtless to a large audience at a Manhattan art gallery, her mastectomy scars fully visible, about the freedom of running "topless 10K's": "We're off! Me, my shirt, and 50,000 people!" In this comic routine she reveals her outrage when, relaxing after the race in the "survivors' café," she is approached by an event official who insists that she either don her shirt or leave. In her saucy memoir, *My One-Night Stand with Cancer,* Katan discusses her familial cancer history and BRCA-positive status as well as plans for an upcoming one-woman show, "Saving Tania's Privates." "If you speak, you survive," she wryly concludes (www.taniaka-tan.com).

Considered as a group, the humorous narratives of Norton, Engelberg, and Wisenberg—along with Sather's blogs, Katan's memoir and YouTube segments, and blog postings by countless other defiant women with breast cancer—constitute feminist activism as well as comic self-expression. Such narratives inform readers that cultural attitudes toward breast cancer have changed since the founding of National Breast Cancer Awareness Month in 1985, since the declaration by the *New York Times* of 1992 as "The Year of the Ribbon," and since the increase in National Cancer Institute funding of research on breast cancer from $155 million in 1992 to $566 million in 2004 (King). Reading humorous narratives can help people living with breast cancer to better cope with illness, suffering, and mortality, since laughter provides a means of deflecting fear and confronting vulnerability. Such narratives invite readers to revel in the knowledge that rebellious laughter "strategically bypasses civility to return us to our body and remind us of our corporeality, momentarily shattering the apparently global imperatives of manners and beauty" (Stott, 86).

5 | New Directions in Breast Cancer Photography
Documenting Women's Post-operative Bodies

Photographic representations of women living with or beyond breast cancer have gained prominence in recent decades due to increasing incidences and heightened public awareness of this disease. Visual breast cancer narratives constitute both documentary projects and dialogic sites of self-construction, for all "selves" are texts to be deciphered, and breast cancer subjectivities can be especially difficult to articulate and decode, given the psychological and cultural weight of this malady. Because of their painful subject matter and iconic power, photographs of women with breast cancer may evoke ambivalence or controversy, as viewers, some of whom may themselves be ill, confront vivid images of scarred, recovering, or deteriorating bodies. In an essay in *Afterimage* Jean Dykstra claims that "given metaphors of the healthy body as 'healthy society' and norms about what is appropriate subject matter for public photographs, autobiographical photographs of bodies marked by disease signify a forceful challenge to codes of representation and cultural ideologies about the female body" (1). Resisting conventional sexualized representations, breast cancer photographs ask readers to reevaluate "standards of beauty and acceptability of images of the female body" and raise important issues of "gender, illness and representation and the construction of the self" (2).

Breast cancer photography made its U.S. mainstream debut on the August 15, 1993, cover of the *New York Times Magazine,* which featured a pale, gaunt woman clad in a striking white dress cut away to reveal the mastectomy scar that dominated her exposed torso. This self-portrait by the photographer and model Matuschka, who was diagnosed with breast cancer in 1991 and underwent a mastectomy that she later deemed unnecessary, was a political gesture that invoked more than a thousand letters to the newspaper, many of them from breast cancer patients (www.matuschka.org). While a majority of these responses were supportive ("Fantastic! A cover girl who looks like me!"), others were critical or even angry: "It's embarrassing!"; "Now everyone knows how I look!" ("Why I Did It"). Entitled *Beauty Out of Damage,* Matuschka's self-portrait introduced an article by Susan Ferraro accompanied by the headline "You Can't Look Away Anymore." This photograph became the most frequently published in the world during 1993 and was nominated for a Pulitzer Prize. "I have always adhered to the philosophy that one should speak and show the truth, because knowledge leads to free will, to choice," explained Matuschka in her essay "Why I Did It." "I hope that my image will convey the idea that a woman with one breast or no breasts is entitled to be looked at and approved of. My message is: 'Don't wait for society to accept you. Have courage to face yourself—the whole package. You become the role model and society will follow'" ("Why I Did It").[1]

Society has indeed followed. As Carol Spiro, president of Ottawa, Canada's branch of Breast Cancer Action (BCA), points out, "Matuschka's cover did more for breast cancer than anyone else in the last twenty-five years" (www.matuschka.org). Although Matuschka's injunction to breast cancer patients to speak out may sound familiar to postmillennial readers, given the current prominence of breast cancer movements in the United States and United Kingdom, her *New York Times* photograph appeared in an era in which activism and research were just beginning to thrive. In 1993 feminist organizations such as the Breast Cancer Fund, the National Breast Cancer Coalition, the Mautner Project, and BCA had recently joined mainstream groups such as Susan G. Komen for the Cure and the American Cancer Society (ACS) in calling for increased research funding and heightened visibility for patients long stigmatized. With the support of the Clinton administration and the U.S. Congress, breast cancer research funding at the National Cancer Institute grew from $155 million in 1992 to $566 million in 2004 (King, ix–xxx). Matuschka's photographs of her mastectomy scar (including *Take This Picture, Like Mother, Like Daughter,* and *Portrait of the Artist as a One-Breasted Activist*) subsequently appeared at breast cancer fund-raising events, and she expressed pride that her self-portraiture broke cultural silence: "If we keep quiet about what cancer does to women's bodies, if we refuse to accept women's bodies in whatever condition they are, we are doing a disservice to womankind" ("Why I Did It").

Since Matuschka was not the first activist to photograph her post-mastectomy body, a brief discussion of earlier representations will contextualize the impact of her *New York Times* cover image. Most historians agree that the earliest image of a one-breasted woman to enter U.S. public space was that of poet Deena Metzger, who in 1977 appeared nude from the waist up, smiling and arms outstretched, on a feminist poster featuring a photograph taken by Hella Hammid.[2] This photograph highlights Metzger's missing right breast, her mastectomy scar covered by a tattooed tree. "There was a fine red line across my chest where a knife entered but now a branch winds about the scar and travels from arm to heart," claims Metzger in an accompanying prose-poem; "I have the body of a warrior who does not kill or wound" (www.deenametzger.com). Although Metzger's photograph is not self-portraiture, she conceptualized the representation of her post-operative body and solicited Hammid to capture this positive image.[3] Lisa Cartwright describes well the differences between the photographic representations of Metzger and Matuschka.

> While Metzger's scar is displayed in a manner that seems to promote its joyous revelation, Matuschka's is artfully lit and framed to emphasis the role of concealment and display in its disclosure. And whereas "The Warrior" puts forth the post-operative woman as a naturally beautiful figure, "Beauty Out of Damage" suggests a concept of beauty whose aesthetic involves an appreciation of the fashioning of the body. (129)

These photographs depict two different breast cancer aesthetics, political stances, and subject formations: Metzger presents herself as healthy and exuberant, her post-mastectomy breast as natural in its unreconstructed state; Matuschka, in contrast, presents her post-operative body as disfigured yet elegant, deserving to be seen.

Matuschka's other important predecessor, British photographer Jo Spence, gained public recognition in the United Kingdom during the 1980s for depicting her breasts pressed down during mammograms and *Marked Up for Amputation*—an ironic photographic title, since she refused the mastectomy her surgeon recommended in favor of lumpectomy. In another photo from this series she wryly labels her left breast *Property of Jo Spence?* With psychologist Rosie Martin, Spence developed techniques of photo-therapy still used to assist patients struggling to counter traumatic experiences. The emphasis in Spence's cancer photographs is neither Metzger's joy nor Matuschka's sobriety but rather a trenchant critique of a sexist culture that fetishizes breasts and a medical system that often objectifies patients.[4] Dykstra notes these differences between the self-portraiture of Matuschka and Spence.

> Many of Matuschka's photographs have a polished, fine arts look about them. Despite their subject matter, they are often beautiful to look at. Spence's photographs, on the other hand, are often snapshot-like, in-your-face documents of her rage and feelings of powerlessness. Matuschka's images suggest a reevaluation of definitions of a beautiful body, and they radiate a kind of pride in a still-beautiful body. Spence's photographs and the pointed, articulate text that accompanies them are interrogations not only of conventions of beauty and the female body, but of codes of representation, constructions of disease, and explorations of identity. Perhaps most significantly, they demand that viewers become aware of the visual codes that construct ideas of gender, sexuality, class, illness and the kind of body that is "fit to be seen." (4)

The Amazonian imagery of Metzger's photograph and poem, the systemic critique of gender and medicalization by Spence, and the resistant yet "beautiful" aesthetic of Matuschka represent a range of activist approaches to documenting women's post-operative bodies in the latter decades of the twentieth century.

Breast cancer photography published in the United States since the mid-1990s has veered away from self-portraiture, as documentary narratives created by a photographer-witness have become the dominant mode of representation. Recent projects have focused on the somatic identities of women combating cancer and have constructed discursive "selves" for both photographer and photographic subjects. In what follows I analyze the cultural work and aesthetic reconfigurations that contemporary breast cancer photographs perform as well as effects their accompanying narratives have had on reader-viewers. As Cartwright notes, "The formation of communities and public cultures on the basis of breast cancer politics entails a reconfiguration of the post-operative female body in public space" (125). Moreover, as a public breast cancer culture has developed, feminist scholars have questioned whether its visual representations are sufficiently diverse. Cartwright, for example, has decried mainstream media emphasis on patients who are white, young, and glamorous, and has argued "in favor of representations that take up the complexities of age and beauty as they pertain to specific groups of women for whom breast cancer is most immediately a concern (women in their fifties and sixties) as well as those women categorically left out of discussions about breast cancer media (for example, black women)" (131). I share these concerns, and in analyzing what breast cancer photography signifies and accomplishes in postmillennial U.S. culture, I consider not only *how* women's post-operative bodies are documented but also *which* women's bodies are represented, and why.

This chapter focuses on five collections of breast cancer photographs that narrate their subjects' experiences of illness, affirm their medicalized bodies, and engage photographer, subjects, and reader-viewers in a complex dialectic of structured looking: Art Myers's *Winged Victory: Altered Images Transcending Breast Cancer* (1996), Amelia Davis's *The First Look* (2000), Jila Nikpay's *Heroines: Transformation in the Face of Breast Cancer* (2006), Amy S. Blackburn's *Caring for Cynthia: A Caregiver's Journey through Breast Cancer* (2008), and Charlee Brodsky and Stephanie Byram's *Knowing Stephanie* (2003). The first three works are anthologies that feature black-and-white images of women of varied ages, races, ethnicities, and body types, identified by either full name or first name. Commentary accompanies the photographs, often the women's own words but sometimes those of photographers, family members, or medical professionals, which serve as textual frames. These photographic narratives might best be characterized as "imagetexts," to use W. J. T. Mitchell's term, collections reliant on "a verbal overlay of relational networks" that inform their cultural inflections (9). In contrast, *Caring for Cynthia* and *Knowing Stephanie* are photo-documentaries, collaborative narratives that trace the illness history of one woman with breast cancer as captured in images taken by her chosen photographer.[5] *Caring for Cynthia* features photographer Amy S. Blackburn's commentary rather than that of Cynthia Ogden, the woman photographed, while *Knowing Stephanie* highlights the ill subject's own words but is framed by photographer Charlee Brodsky's preface and a biographical essay by Jennifer Matesa. These collections bring visibility to breast cancer patients by exploring their post-surgical embodiment and chronicling their hard-won subjectivities. They challenge hegemonic cultural definitions of beauty and femininity, and invite reader-viewers to witness images of women's somatic suffering, resilience, or resistance. Despite these strengths, however, several of the narratives heterosexualize the breast cancer subject, feature hyperfeminine images, employ sentimental discourses, and/or emphasize a "mindless triumphalism" that risks dishonoring those who have died of this disease (Ehrenreich, 53). Since *The First Look* and *Knowing Stephanie* avoid these pitfalls, it is instructive to consider how so.

Transcendent Discourses in *Winged Victory*

In *Family Frames: Photography, Narrative, and Postmemory* Marianne Hirsch reminds readers that although photography's primary function since the nineteenth century has been the documentation of family life, "multiple looks circulate in the photograph's production, reading, and description"; familial photographs made public, that is to say, invite new ideologies of spectatorship (1). The context for Hirsch's observation is her reflection on Roland Barthes's analysis in *Camera Lucida* of his most highly revered family heirloom, the so-called winter garden photograph taken of his recently deceased mother when she was a child. For Barthes, this photograph's *punctum*—the sting of recognition, "that accident which pricks me (but also bruises me, is poignant to me)"—lies in the familiar expression on the face of the girl who would later give birth to him (Barthes, 27). This jolt of recognition explains the photograph's emotional resonance, a resonance that Barthes considered comprehensible only for himself as grieving son; he thus withholds the photograph from his reader's view. Hirsch extrapolates from Barthes's analysis to consider familial photographs more broadly through interpretations that rest on what he terms the *studium,* "the contextual, cultural narrative that helps one read a photograph" (Hirsch, 3). Competing cultural narratives evoke shifting interpretations; hence Hirsch's claim that whenever photographic portraits are publicly scrutinized, multiple looks circulate.

Hirsch's caveat is relevant to Art Myers's *Winged Victory* because that collection's stated impetus is familial experience, and one featured subject is the photographer's wife, Stephanie Myers. As a specialist in preventive medicine, Myers explains in his preface, he has "many times had the sobering responsibility of delivering the news of a cancer diagnosis to patients and their loved ones" (np). Yet when his sister was diagnosed with breast cancer in her thirties (she subsequently died of the disease), and when his wife faced surgery some years later, Myers was "not prepared for the overwhelming effect that breast cancer in two close family members would have on my life" (np). The narrative subjectivity that Myers constructs is thus medically authoritative but experientially naive. A fine-arts photographer as well as a physician, Myers expresses hope that this project will "show that a woman's fundamental nature is not dependent on anything external; the loss of part or all of her breast is not a threat to her being" (np). Although his assumptions regarding "a woman's fundamental nature" may sound essentialist from a feminist perspective, Myers challenges mainstream U.S. media for "bombard[ing]" viewers with "messages of centerfolds, push-up bras and silicone implants" that contribute to some men's discomfort with amputated breasts and may exacerbate the fears of women with breast cancer that their "body image, femininity, and sexuality" are at risk (np).

Three photographs in *Winged Victory* offer images of post-operative women that challenge conventional assumptions of disfiguration or victimization. The first of these, captioned *Sisterhood,* presents a chain of linked photos in which diverse women display their nude breasts, unreconstructed or reconstructed, and face the camera, hands outstretched toward one another. The accompanying narrative written by one of the subjects, Dani, advances the theme of strength in community: "The gift of a lifetime came to me from the sisterhood of strangers who reached out to share their metamorphic journey from breast cancer victim to woman of substance" (Myers, np). Praising Myers for realizing that if his subjects would "openly expose their scars," that act would "make acceptance a visible and essential concomitant of beauty," Dani claims that subjects found common purpose during this project: "One by one we came to see our involvement as a way to change perceptions." An additional benefit for the women was "an enhanced sense of self-esteem and pride in their bodies" (Myers, np). The *punctum* of this photograph arguably occurs through paradox: the vulnerability of the women's scarred breasts, the strength of their gazes. The photograph's *studium* lies in the culturally inflected knowledge that these women—old and young; black, white, and Asian; de-breasted or newly re-breasted—visually instantiate the experiences of thousands of post-operative women. *Sisterhood* constructs a visible link among breast cancer subjects who implicitly invite reciprocal others to share their illness narratives.

Painted Ladies, the only color image in *Winged Victory,* portrays three smiling women whose de-breasted or one-breasted chests have been decorated.[6] As revealed in Dani's commentary, the subjects and the artist chose the imagery that would adorn each breast and the pose each woman would assume. Dani, a bodysurfer who enjoys defying the law by surfing topless, chose to pose as "the wink," her right breast painted as an eye with staring pupil, her breastless left side surrounded by eye-

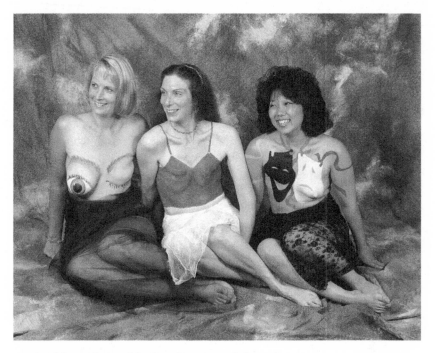

Art Myers, *Painted Ladies.* Courtesy of the artist.

lashes that give the illusion of winking. Carol, who underwent a bilateral mastectomy, was "transformed into a woman with cleavage in a beautiful blue camisole," while Susan, "with theatrical flair, became comedy and tragedy, with each intentionally reversed so that the comedy mask appeared over the mastectomy scar" (Myers, np). Post-surgical breasts have sported tattoos and body art for decades, but this photo further subverts the cultural script of breast cancer as tragic by engaging women's post-operative bodies as humorous artistic canvases. In addition, the photograph and accompanying text pay homage to the women's bonds: "From Carol to Dani to Susan, we each served as mentor and friend to each other when we were diagnosed. Years later we celebrated our friendships in living color" (Myers, np).

A third photograph, *Lisa with Barbell,* presents in semi-profile a short-haired, bare-breasted woman gazing at the impressively flexed muscle of her right arm while holding an enormous free weight in her left hand. Although her breasts are asymmetrical—the right breast is large and unscarred, the left smaller, scarred, and muscular—her arms appear symmetrical, their muscles well developed. Lisa's accompanying testimony emphasizes agency and strength, doctor-patient collaboration, and pleasure in her distinctive bodily contours.

> *I've made changes, reshaped my body with the use of free weights and aerobics over the last twelve years. And the surgeon made his changes when he removed my breast. A bit odd, perhaps, but I enjoy the change in that when I look at my chest where he removed my breast, I can truly appreciate and enjoy the shape and lines that I have added to my body over the years with the weights. The contrast is appealing to me, a soft breast on one side and a hard "pec" on the other.* (Myers, np)

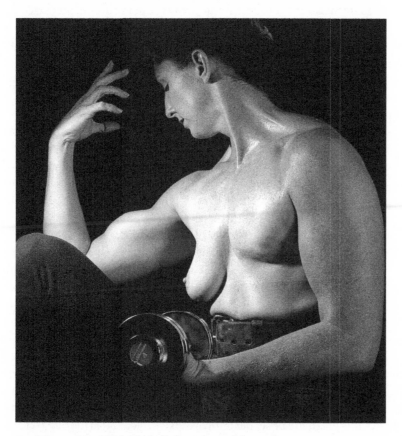

Art Myers, *Lisa With Barbell.* Courtesy of the artist.

Lisa's comments reflect a breast cancer aesthetic that celebrates hybrid embodiment, while the photograph highlights her transgendered appearance. This imagetext challenges the dominant cultural narrative that women who undergo breast cancer surgery inevitably strive to regain their "lost" femininity.

The phrase *altered images,* which appears in the book's subtitle, addresses an intriguing aspect of several Myers photographs reliant on montage, most notably the untitled cover image of a one-breasted woman whose lower body has become a gnarled tree trunk and whose shoulders and head have morphed into leafy branches. Myers's use of tree imagery to convey the strength of post-mastectomy women recalls the poem that accompanied publication of the Hammid photograph of Metzger, but his photograph draws upon surrealist traditions to present the breast cancer body as mysterious—a theme reinforced by the talismanic necklace that the woman-tree wears, a bird whose feathers are attached to a wreath of vines and berries. Any potential this image might have to move beyond exoticism is unfortunately diminished by the Maria Marrocchino poem that glosses it, "Sometimes a Leaf Will Fall before Autumn," which features predictable lines such as "Sometimes true beauty can never be captured" (Myers, np).[7]

Despite many engaging photographs, *Winged Victory* at times romanticizes, sentimentalizes, and heterosexualizes women with breast cancer and thereby undercuts its subversive potential. The tendency to glorify hegemonic femininity appears most notably in *Stephanie,* which features the photographer's wife clad in a long, sweeping dress that drapes her arms and shoulders, gathers at the waist, and opens to reveal her breasts, which appear at first glance unmarked by surgery. A closer look, however, reveals what the accompanying text confirms, that her right breast is reconstructed; a scar is barely visible, and the right nipple has a slightly different color and texture from the left. *"My breast and right arm took quite a beating after the lympectomy, lymphadenectomy, surgery, radiation and radioactive implants,"* she explains. *"Over time my breast has again become fairly symmetrical"* (Myers, np). Although an unsettling medical narrative clearly exists, neither Art nor Stephanie Myers tells that story. Both the *studium* of this photograph and its subject's commentary configure breast reconstruction as a means of producing a highly desirable symmetry—a concept reinforced by the photo's glamour-shot layout and Stephanie's dramatic pose, head thrown back, cloaked arms outstretched, bare breasts thrust forward in an unsettling representation of feminine beauty fetishized.

Part of the tension between conventional and subversive representation that characterizes Myers's photographs lies in his emphasis on the Winged Victory of Samothrace, the famous classical Greek statue of an armless woman with exposed breasts, draped thighs, and wings attached to her shoulders that graces the entry chamber of the Louvre in Paris. The book's foreword, written by physician David Spiegel, describes this statue as a powerful representation of "female strength transcending the ravages of time," a strength parallel to that of the women photographed by Myers, who "say 'Here I am.' They are redefining their beauty: breasts missing, reconstructed, they present their bodies and themselves with humor, sadness, vulnerability, honesty. . . . They do not hide their loss; they transcend it" (Spiegel in Myers, foreword, np). With the exception of *Lisa with Barbell* and *Painted Ladies,* the romantic theme of feminine beauty lost and regained dominates *Winged Victory,* as exemplified by Dani's claim that all of the women photographed "retain the classic notion of beauty" despite their "imperfections" (Myers, np). A discourse of transcendence likewise recurs, as the collection's subtitle and Siegel's foreword reveal. Such rhetoric also dominates the Marrocchino poems that punctuate the text: in "Venus" she describes a single-breasted woman *"who transcends humanity / with magical grace"*; in "Transcendence" she rhapsodizes over a photograph of a man's and a woman's hands clasped across a scarred breast (Myers, np).

The term *transcendence* signifies a breast cancer sublime that becomes problematic in *Winged Victory* by implying that survivors experience rapture in ways that other humans do not. Images that link cancer and its survival to discourses of the sublime occur in many poems by Marrocchino, with their references to the "rainbow gardens," "golden skies," "evening vines," "emerald hands," "rapturous lands," and "cosmic wings" that one encounters during or after breast cancer. One romantic lyric even contains the word *sublime:* the photograph accompanying "My Hands, My Body" shows a woman's fingers caressing her breasts, celebrating *"a body like a sublime cloud that drifts into the cool skies"* (Myers, np). At times a triumphalist rhetoric dominates this collection, reinforced by romantic imagery, claims of transcendence, and the word *victory* in its title. As Barbara Ehrenreich has argued, "mindless triumphalism . . . denigrates the dead and the dying. Did we who live 'fight' harder than those who have died?" (53).[8] The triumphant discourse of *Winged Victory* risks implying that women who live years after having cancer are winners while those who die have lost a macabre competition.

Heterosexual romance sometimes becomes a distracting focus of Myers's narrative, since six out of twenty photographs present post-mastectomy women posing with their male partners. In these images all of the women bare their chests, as do three of the men (wittily); the other three men are presented as fully clothed companions. Perhaps the most romantic of these photos is *Carol and Dick,* a portrait of a middle-aged, breastless woman carrying an elegant tray of glowing candles; along-side is her distinguished, white-bearded partner dressed in black. Both subjects gaze soberly at the camera as the accompanying narrative pro-claims their mutual devotion; Carol describes Dick as *"my soul-mate,"* while he calls her *"this lean, flat-chested beauty"* who *"would be my salva-tion"* (Myers, np). Since Myers's collection depicts no lesbian partners, the effect is to foreground heterosexuality as a normative force that al-lows cancer to be transcended. Myers's preface explains this emphasis, since he argues that women's anxiety at a breast cancer diagnosis quickly transforms into a fear of "diminished femininity," a concern he seems to view as ubiquitous despite some of his subjects' claims to the contrary. He describes scenarios he has witnessed as a physician between patients and their male partners—admittedly realistic in some cases, yet unfor-tunately stereotypical—in which "a partner withdraws a hand to avoid touching a scar where once was a graceful curve"; too often, he suggests, cancer makes "lovers draw apart, an absent breast now a barrier to their intimacy" (Myers, preface, np). To be fair, Myers rightly decries such acts of rejection and celebrates "the persistence of a woman's beauty, strength and femaleness in all of its complexity, even after the transforming ex-perience of breast cancer"—but the phrase "even after" implies that res-toration is hard for a post-operative woman to achieve without an erotic bond with a supportive man (np).

In its emphasis on classical beauty, romantic imagery, transcendence, and heteronormativity, Myers's photographic documentation of women's breast cancer bodies can only be interpreted as culturally hegemonic. However, his inclusion of photographs that foreground racial, gender, and age diversity and present women's post-operative bodies playfully makes *Winged Victory* an important work of visual testimony.

Feminist Discourses in *The First Look*

In viewing photographic representations of women's breast cancer bodies, both dominant and alternative cultural ideologies inevitably come into play. As Hirsch points out in *Family Frames*, "The structure of looking is reciprocal: photographer and viewer collaborate in the reproduction of ideology. . . . Eye and screen are the very elements of ideology: our expectations circumscribe and determine what we show and what we see" (7). This critical insight provides a useful point of departure for analyzing the ideologies that circulate in representations of women's post-surgical bodies from Amelia Davis's *The First Look*. Like Myers, Davis undertook her photographic project for familial reasons; her mother, one of twenty-six featured subjects, was diagnosed with breast cancer at sixty-seven and felt "unprepared for the way she would look after a modified radical mastectomy—her only option—and how she would feel about herself" (xiii). Since the only representations of post-mastectomy women's bodies that Davis's mother could locate in 1993 were technical drawings of thin, flat scars, she felt betrayed after surgery when her scars bore no resemblance to those depicted in medical journals. "I decided then that no woman should ever feel this way," explains Davis in her preface (xiii). For Davis and her collaborators, realistic representation of women's post-operative bodies takes precedence over altered images; hence the photographer presents her subjects relaxing in their homes rather posing before studio lights. Having rejected a rhetoric of transcendence, Davis features instead a feminist approach to the structure of looking—a reciprocal collaboration among subjects, photographer, and audience.

In one respect, however, Davis's photographs are problematic from a feminist perspective, for the subjects in *The First Look* are disturbingly faceless; only their torsos are depicted. To be sure, Davis offers a thoughtful rationale for this decision.

I chose not to include the women's faces in these photographs for several reasons. In the beginning some women requested that their faces not be shown, and as time went on, I realized that their faces were unnecessary, even an impediment, to this project. The photographs are intended to let women see exactly what mastectomies, various types of reconstructive surgery, and lumpectomies look like, and I did not want to take the reader's attention away from that. Because today's society places so much emphasis on looks, the faces distracted from this purpose. (xiii–xiv)

Despite Davis's argument that concerns for privacy, aesthetic consider-ations, and a critique of social norms regarding female beauty informed her choice, the ideological message of faceless images of post-operative women arguably endorses concealment and fragmentation. Without depiction of the eyes through which a subject meets photographer and camera, she cannot participate fully in reciprocal looking. As Matuschka once asked a photographer whom she had refused permission to repre-sent her body without showing her face, "Why can't you have the head in the picture and still look great, just because part of your body has been removed?" (www.matuschka.org). Although Davis clearly hopes to empower her subjects, her collection risks reproducing the dominant cultural ideology that it is acceptable to show breasts without making visible the whole woman.

That said, *The First Look* brings many strengths to its representation of women's breast cancer bodies, especially a diversity of age, race, body type, reconstruction status, and life writing. The women photographed range in age from twenty-five to seventy-six; more than half are over forty-five. Most photographs present the women alone; three appear with a child, one woman with her dog (also a cancer survivor). Although Davis captures no images of women who self-identify as lesbians, neither does she foreground heterosexuality in her collection as Myers does. Five of Davis's photographic subjects identify themselves as African Ameri-can and two as Asian American; several comment on their working-class identities. In her preface Davis affirms her commitment to diversity of representation.

It is important to me, not only as a photographer but also as a woman, to try to represent all women in this book because breast cancer does not discriminate. This disease affects women of all ages, all ethnic groups, and all socioeconomic backgrounds. Every woman has a voice and every woman should be heard. (xiv)

The women Davis photographs do offer a remarkable variety of testimo-nies. Wanda, for example, an African American woman photographed with her young son in the background, reveals that she discovered her breast tumor at twenty-eight, shortly after the birth of her seventh child, while enrolled in a drug treatment program. Despite having no health insurance, Wanda obtained a mastectomy that was followed by eighteen grueling months of chemotherapy, access to breast cancer support groups that she deemed vital, and a new career as a milliner: "Going through cancer, I had picked up a little skill of making hats—fashion hats. It was something I wanted to give back to the community. I lost all my hair, so I got into hats—I thought I could pass it on to other women" (Davis, 33). Equally memorable is the story of Marleen, a forty-eight-year-old Portuguese Pacific Islander who reports having endured five operations—lumpectomy, modified radical mastectomy, and multiple reconstruction surgeries—and includes in her narrative an excerpt from her poem "Silent Soldier—Invisible Amputee" (Davis, 63). Out of their breast cancer experience Wanda and Marleen construct powerful subjectivities that reader-viewers are invited to witness.

The First Look offers equal representation to reconstructed and unreconstructed breasts; it also depicts women's arms with and without lymphedema, the debilitating swelling that often accompanies the removal of lymph nodes after breast cancer surgery. Shevra, for instance, a forty-year-old woman pictured with her reconstructed breast grasped by the infant daughter she adopted after treatment rendered her infertile, proffers a tightly bandaged left arm and identifies her lymphedema as chronic. She also conveys her motivation for undergoing reconstruction.

> At the time I did not really question having reconstructive surgery, I just assumed I would do it. I went through three operations within the first year because I thought they would put me back together again. They helped me put off my reaction to losing my breast, but eventually that caught up with me. What I have now works fine under clothes and I'm used to it, but it's not a breast and it doesn't resemble what I lost. I even had to have cosmetic surgery on my healthy breast so that it would look more like my reconstructed "breast." If I had it to do over, I don't know whether I would choose reconstructive surgery. (Davis, 1)

Some of Davis's photographic subjects affirm their choice of reconstruction, while others recount complications, regret their decision, or report having never considered it. Noemi, twenty-eight, expresses pride in now having "the prettiest breast in the whole world" and relief at not "having

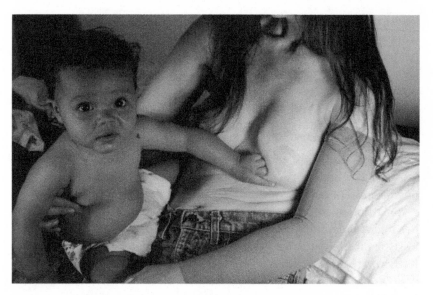

Amelia Davis, *Shevra*. Courtesy of the artist.

to worry anymore about a prosthesis sagging or shifting," whereas Rachel, also twenty-eight, rejects both prosthesis and reconstruction, lamenting that a "'do-nothing' option is one seldom discussed by doctors" (Davis, 22, 5). Although *The First Look* endorses neither reconstruction nor its alternative, the unreconstructed breasts on display slightly outnumber the reconstructed; this balance reflects the fact that in 2000, when this book was published, fewer than 40 percent of U.S. women with breast cancer chose reconstruction.[9] The collection does contain a concluding essay by a plastic surgeon, Loren Eshkanazi, who discusses options available to women who choose breast reconstruction, from saline or silicone implants to TRAM flap procedures; also featured is an array of medical photographs of women's breasts prior to and following reconstructive surgery. A second medically informative essay, written by registered nurse Saskia Thiadens, explains causes and treatments for lymphedema and likewise contains illustrative medical photographs.

Another feminist aspect of Davis's photographs and her subjects' testimonies is their representation of post-surgical scars as insignia of resistance. Women who have refused reconstruction are particularly vocal on this topic: Marge, for instance, describes her post-mastectomy scar as a "badge of courage"; for Rachel it represents a "battle wound," for Ruth a "battle scar" (Davis, 27, 5, 50). This emphasis challenges hegemonic no-

tions of femininity by codifying scars as symbols of strength and affirming their capacity for beauty. As physician Nancy Snyderman claims in
her foreword to *The First Look,* "the human body is its own art form," and
"bodies with scars have not left the art behind" (x). Marge endorses this

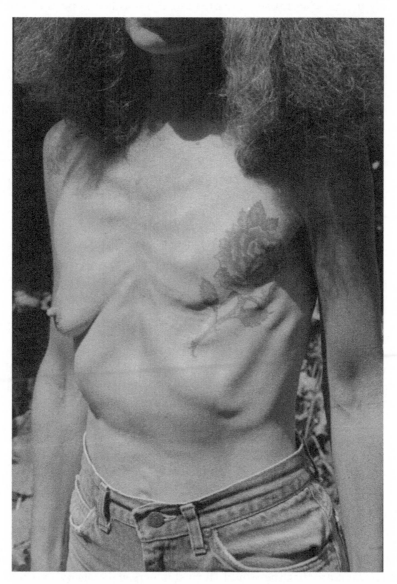

Amelia Davis, *Andrée.* Courtesy of the artist.

perspective: "I am a beautiful person inside and out. . . . We all have scars, but some are more visible than others" (Davis, 27). Tattoos and scars converge in some photographic representations, a trend that began in the 1980s, after widespread circulation of the Metzger poster of the tree tattoo that covers her missing breast, and has intensified in postmillennial culture, with its pervasive emphasis on body piercings and artful tattooing.[10] Davis's photograph of the tattooed breast of her subject Andrée, for example, foregrounds its flowery artistry. As Andrée's commentary affirms, her tattoo serves as a form of bodily and spiritual affirmation: "My left breast has transformed itself into a red rose—sacred—which grows in my dreams" (Davis, 71). Although several of Davis's photographic subjects express discomfort with their mastectomy scars, most agree with Snyderman that scars "mark the trail, the passage taken" through the breast cancer continuum (Davis, x).

In her preface Davis states her goal of providing accurate information and feminist support for women facing breast surgery.

> With this book in hand, women can eliminate their preconceived images of what breast cancer looks like and replace them with realities. Having visual representations of these realities removes the mystery and perhaps the fear. When a woman is diagnosed with breast cancer, I hope she will pick up this book . . . and feel comfort in knowing that she is not alone. (xiv–xv)

In the comments that accompany their photographs several participants make explicit the political agenda that led to their appearance in this project. Merijane, for example, whose one-breasted image appears on the book's cover, challenges environmental myopia.

> There is still no cure for breast cancer. All the technology intended to make us "beautiful" after we have been cut, radiated, and filled with toxic chemicals does not alter that fact. Until the *real* causes of this disease—the human-made, environmental causes—are addressed with commitment and sincerity, the word *prevention* holds no meaning. (Davis, 60)

Equally outspoken is Raven Light, a San Francisco activist who decided after diagnosis that she would "turn this personal tragedy into public awareness."

Since then I have bared my de-breast in a fierce political stance. Breast cancer has been hidden under heavy layers of shame, guilt, and puffs of cotton stuffed inside empty bras for too many decades. I choose to use my body to put a face on this hideous disease—to stand tall, placing the humanness of breast cancer in everyone's line of sight. My breast and de-breast are seen at parades, on postcards, on the walls of museums, in newspapers and magazines across this country and as far as Zaire. (Davis, 53–54)

Overall, *The First Look* challenges viewers to gaze openly at women's post-operative bodies, bear attentive witness to their narratives of illness and recovery, and consider engaging in breast cancer activism.

Spiritual Discourses in *Heroines*

An Iranian expatriate photographer, poet, and teacher drawn to the topic of breast cancer through workshops on body image that she led, Jila Nikpay began a collaborative project to document the spiritual journeys of Minneapolis women who had contracted this disease. Between 2002 and 2004 she interviewed twenty-one women from thirty-three to seventy-three—African American, Arab, American Indian, and Caucasian—who were willing to be photographed and share their cancer narratives with viewers. Nikpay's aesthetic strategy of offering swaths of black-and-white cloth that her photographic subjects could use to wrap, drape, conceal, or reveal their bodies allowed her to "transform the veil from an icon of body repression into an artistic tool" (Klefsted). To complement the photographs in *Heroines*, Nikpay includes prose-poems that capture the emotional flavor of each woman's cancer experience, as mediated through the lens of the interview. The primary advantages of this methodology are the photographic subjects' creative use of cloth to conceal or reveal their breast cancer bodies and the vivid imagery that Nikpay's poetry invokes. Disadvantages include the absence of the women's own voices and the presence of sentimental discourses of heroism and hope.

In her preface to *Heroines* Nikpay describes her photo-narrative project in spiritual terms: "My subjects have realized that beyond this hinterland of suffering lies a body of water in which the spirit caresses their souls and heals their wounds" (9). Metaphors of geography abound here alongside religious, mystical, and medical imagery of pain and healing. Such metaphors anticipate the spiritual motifs that Nikpay engages in her poems, in which she represents Islamic, Christian, Native American, and Buddhist imagery. For example, both the beauty of Islamic traditions and the restrictiveness of conservative Arab gender norms are implicit in the photographic representation of Hend Al-Mansour, age forty when she was diagnosed with breast cancer while studying in the United States. In this photograph Al-Mansour uses a white cotton cloth as a form of hijab to wrap her body and head so that only her face is visible; she gazes directly at the photographer with an expression at once melancholy and defiant. Nikpay's poetic monologue captures the isolation that Al-Mansour experienced in having breast cancer abroad: "Shall I tell my family? / No. For an Arab woman / Body is perfect or else" (49). This poem rejects cultural fetishizing of idealized female embodiment yet depicts its subject's fear that her cancerous body will be stigmatized. Still, Al-Mansour allows her shrouded body to be revealed, her mediated story told. The final stanza of Nikpay's poem positions Al-Mansour as a transgressive artist who embraces the vitality and imaginative energy to "build . . . / Imaginary worlds" (49). Together, Nikpay's poem and the photographic image of Al-Mansour create a narrative of cultural resistance and spiritual transformation.

Christian imagery appears in several poems from *Heroines,* as Nikpay alludes to God's work, the children of God, and Christ's suffering on the cross. The photograph of Betty Sanders, a fifty-year-old African American woman twice diagnosed with breast cancer, recalls the dignified posture of Rosa Parks following her initiation of the Montgomery bus boycotts in 1955. Standing erect in semi-profile, Sanders gazes resolutely toward the heavens, hands spread at her side; she wears a black cloak elegantly as a strapless gown with a shawl covering one shoulder, an improvised garment that partially reveals her breasts. The speaker in Nikpay's poem admits having changed from her cancer ordeal and alludes to the presence of a tattoo that the image does not reveal: "A big red rose / Hides my scars / And reminds me: / My work is / God's work" (41). Here Nikpay employs Christian imagery to invest her subject's body and life purpose with spiritual authority. A related imagery informs the poem for Jymme Golden, diagnosed at thirty-six with breast cancer that required a bilateral mastectomy. Her lower body wrapped in a white toga, Golden poses like a Greek sculpture with head in graceful profile, right arm outstretched, fingertips holding a sheer veil that edges her left shoulder. The accompanying poem employs Christian imagery to describe Golden's surgical incision as forming "a memorable cross / Across my chest" (19). After celebrating Golden's new calling as a massage therapist, the poem ends with images of transfiguration: "In body, mind, and soul, / I am transformed" (19). In this instance Nikpay uses Christian symbolism to depict a subject at peace with her breastlessness.

Native American spirituality occurs in the Nikpay poem that accompanies her photograph of Clara NiiSka, presented in dignified semi-profile—gray hair braided, hands folded across her chest, body draped in a black cloak whose V-shaped neckline reveals a puckered scar where her right breast used to be. Fifty-two when diagnosed with breast cancer, NiiSka initially responded by feeling "exiled from my tribe" and determined to join her late husband: "I lay on my husband's grave. / I accepted my death" (35). A friend's gift of poetry inspired NiiSka to move through grief with a renewed purpose: "To guard the oral traditions / Of my people" (35). Nikpay's poem uses simple diction to depict the speaker's mission of cultural protection.

Buddhist imagery occurs in *Heroines* in the first of two photographic portraits of Sarah Wovcha, thirty-two. In the initial image her head is bald, her gaze otherworldly, her body shrouded in a white pleated robe.[11] Wovcha's hands touch her face and neck protectively; her demeanor recalls that of Zen monks engaged in meditative walking. Nikpay's poem offers the brevity of haiku: "I closed my eyes to death / Imagining life. / Dreams were my medicine" (13). In a newspaper article about the *Heroines* project, Wovcha explains that she hesitated to be photographed: "Before the session I was thinking, 'I can't tell my story to people. They don't want to hear.'" But working with Nikpay gave her strength: "The project was an invitation not to hide what was happening, but the opposite: to show people all the pieces of the illness. Not to put a wig on. Not to put on a happy face" (Miller). Wovcha's emphasis on visibility suggests a feminist element to this project that does not appear in the text of *Heroines,* which emphasizes spiritual growth over political agency. Nikpay does evince feminist consciousness, however, in interviews in which she discusses problematic attitudes toward embodiment in both Iranian and U.S. societies: "To me, Iranian culture veils the body and American culture veils the soul. I have two different realities, and neither celebrates women" (Miller). The second photograph of Wovcha portrays its subject, pregnant and radiant, curly hair restored, gazing resolutely at the camera. The accompanying poem affirms the power of maternity for a young woman who feared she might never conceive, yet did: "Against all odds / I gave birth. / We are four now" (15). Wovcha explains in an interview that the *Heroines* project gave her peace of mind: "Now I don't care if I have breasts. I don't care if I have hair. I feel content to move through the world and feel the sunshine and rain. And I feel beautiful if my body can be a recipient of those experiences" (Miller).

Nikpay's collection can be critiqued for its engagement of sentimental discourses of "caressing the soul" and "creating a chorus of hope" (9). Although an emphasis on hope may appeal to reader-viewers, as S. Lochlann Jain argues in "Be Prepared," such sentimental discourses risk marginalizing patients who cannot face cancer hopefully.

> Tropes of hope, survivorship, battling, and positive attitude are fed to people post-diagnosis as if they were at the helm of a ship in known waters, not along stormy and uncharted shores. And yet, so little of cancer science, patient experience, or survival statistics seems to provide backing for the ubiquitous calls for hope in the popular cultures of cancer. . . . Such cultural venues as marches for hope, research funding and directions, pharmaceutical interests, survivor rhetoric, and hospital ads constitute not distinct cultural phenomena, but overlap to form a broad hegemony of ways that cancer is talked about and that in turn diminish the ways that cancer culture can be inhabited and spoken about. (170–71)

Jain's argument is useful for evaluating Nikpay's discourse, which moves from suffering to hope without always acknowledging the costs of this disease. In addition, discourses of hope can merge into triumphalist rhetoric. While Nikpay claims in interviews to dislike the term *survivor,* and indeed the word does not appear in *Heroines,* she at times implies that her photographic subjects have triumphed: "We're not saying, 'You survived.' No! You are a heroine. You went beyond" (Miller). Although may be true that the *Heroines* subjects are exceptional women engaged in what Ehrenreich wryly terms "spiritual upward mobility," the implication of Nikpay's rhetoric is that heroines trump terrified women with breast cancer, not to mention those who have died of it (Ehrenreich, 49).

To be sure, the problems suggested by Nikpay's discourses of heroism and hope arise in many other forms of breast cancer culture. As Jackie Stacey notes in *Teratologies,* "masculine" cancer narratives often deify male oncologists and surgeons as "heroic men of medicine" who "save women from the horrors of their own bodies" (11). Stacey also critiques alternative discourses that represent patients as required to heal themselves, thus "generating fantasies of heroic recoveries and miracle cures" that fail to challenge master narratives but instead reposition an ill woman as "masculinised hero" (10–11). Stacey's theory clarifies that heroic cancer discourses such as Nikpay's risk privileging triumphant quest myths while disregarding unsuccessful questers.

Despite these problems, *Heroines* affirms its subjects' post-operative bodies in compelling ways. Participants have testified as to the project's power in their lives; in Wovcha's words, "Cancer can close people down or open them up. . . . I was moving down the path of it closing me down until I met with Jila. That day in front of the camera, I found that I didn't have any fear" (Miller). In addition, several *Heroines* exhibitions, along with related workshops held in Minnesota between 2006 and 2008, initiated community conversations about breast cancer. Nikpay argues that such dialogues foster intercultural exchange. As an Iranian who now lives in America, she explains, she has often "walked a tightrope" in her life and art: "Dialogue is essential for this type of work because it needs to be decoded and in that process a deeper understanding of cultures can take place" (Klefsted).

Caregiving Discourses in *Caring for Cynthia*

The most engaging aspect of *Caring for Cynthia* might likewise be viewed as a limitation: while its photographs depict the struggles of Cynthia Ogden, the focal breast cancer patient, its narrative is written by photographer Amy S. Blackburn, Cynthia's best friend and primary caregiver. Although Blackburn's approach brings attention to the strains and rewards of care providers, readers might wish that Cynthia's words had been included. Blackburn's approach raises the question of effects on reader-viewers when the visual post-operative "self" differs from the narrative subjectivity that a text constructs. Do we see Cynthia through her own eyes, Amy's, both women's? Blackburn presents this project as collaborative, explaining that it began on the evening of Cynthia's diagnosis, when she tearfully asked Blackburn, "Can you take a picture of me tonight—just the way I am right now?" (2). Blackburn did so, and this photograph inaugurated their documentary exploration.[12] Early in her narrative Blackburn describes that initial photograph: "I saw a stoic woman in a black sports bra and polyester running pants, void of expression. Cynthia cried, then regained her composure. In the seven exposures I created that evening, there was already evidence of Cynthia's courage surfacing" (2). Subsequent photographs document her vulnerability as well as strength, especially images that expose her post-mastectomy chest in a manner resistant to "discourses that constitute the diseased body as 'other'" (Dykstra, 4).

Empathy, immediacy, and awareness lie at the heart of this photographic documentary, which offers neither an homage to the beauty of women's post-operative bodies (as *Winged Victory* does), a celebration of bodily diversity (as *The First Look* does), nor a narrative of spiritual transformation (as *Heroines* does). Instead, Blackburn's color photographs and self-reflective commentary lend an intimate quality to her documentation. Her subject, Cynthia Ogden, is white, middle-class, blonde, young, athletic, Christian, and successful, characteristics that describe Amy Blackburn as well; hence no racial-ethnic nor age diversity is evident, and neither marital status nor sexual orientation is mentioned. In her narrative Blackburn foregrounds the need for heightened breast cancer awareness: even though Cynthia was a physician specializing in internal medicine and Amy a registered nurse, neither felt prepared to confront this disease personally. Blackburn explains in her preface that despite years of nursing, she did not recognize the depth of patient anxiety or the centrality of familial support until she accompanied Cynthia through cancer. While Cynthia's story is the narrative's focus, Blackburn makes an admission about herself.

> Another—unexpected—narrative developed during Cynthia's journey, a narrative pertinent to a caregiver: I, the caregiver, changed through my caring for Cynthia.
>
> Breast cancer affected me. It scared me. I developed sympathetic symptoms in response to what Cynthia was physically experiencing: I felt a heavy ache in my chest after the mastectomy and an intermittent low level of nausea in the months that I cared for her. (Preface)

Although Blackburn praises the caregiving community that sustained Cynthia and herself, her narrative remains dyadic—or triadic, since reader-viewers come to feel that we too know Amy and Cynthia.

This perception is rooted in the sense of immediacy that accompanies photographs taken during Ogden's diagnostic, surgical, and post-operative procedures.[13] Blackburn's narrative positions reader-viewers as attentive witnesses to the process that breast cancer catalyzes, not merely to its aftermath. Organized chronologically, *Caring for Cynthia* follows its subject's medical trajectory in a linear fashion, beginning with "She Told Me," a chapter that presents the results of Cynthia's biopsy. Subsequent chapters document her decision to undergo a bilateral mastectomy due to family history (her mother is a breast cancer survivor), her consultation with a plastic surgeon about breast reconstruction (which she subsequently rejects), and Amy's account of Cynthia's surgery and recovery. The hospital narrative is accompanied by a melancholy photo of the gowned patient in bed and holding a medical chart labeled "Ogden, Cynthia. NUC. MED."; a later grim photograph depicts Cynthia sleeping after surgery, swollen and drugged. In this instance Blackburn's narrative presents her own emotional landscape, however, not that of Cynthia: "Did I answer her questions correctly? Do we have everything we will need at the hospital? Am I doing everything right? Is there something I should say?" (18).

Two early chapters foreground the alienation from their post-operative bodies that many women feel. In "Seeing Her Body for the First Time" Blackburn chronicles Cynthia's examination of her post-surgical body, a bandage covering her incisions. Blackburn's photograph of the patient's tentative unwrapping of surgical tape, entitled *Bandage,* reveals Ogden's anxious expression. Amy's narrative and Cynthia's concave chest may create in reader-viewers a sense of bearing uneasy witness to an intimate moment: "Each layer of wrapping had more dried blood the closer she got to the incision. Once the incision was exposed, she looked up to the mirror and then turned to me. There was silence. There were no tears" (30). In a subsequent chapter, "The Drains," Blackburn depicts the complications with fluid release that delay removal of Ogden's post-operative drains, "one of the most intolerable aspects of breast cancer for Cynthia," who eventually insists that doctors remove the drains prematurely (32). This removal causes chest pain due to internal fluid accumulation; hence Cynthia must visit her surgeon's office every few days to have the fluid removed by needle, a process documented photographically in a gruesome shot of her scarred torso from which a bulbous tube snakes, as a technician's gloved hands insert a needle into her flesh. As the collection's most medically graphic images, these two photographs raise important somatic and psychological issues of how women confront their post-operative bodies.

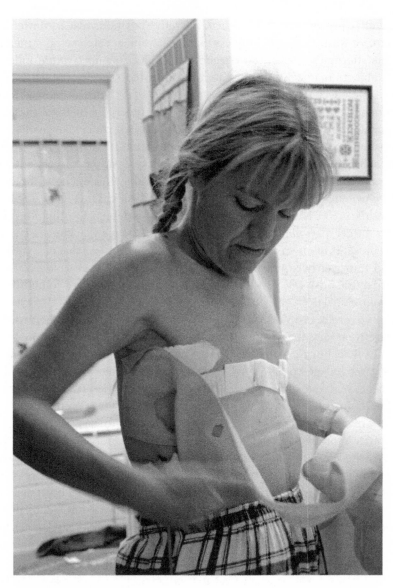

Amy S. Blackburn, *Bandage*. © Amy S. Blackburn.

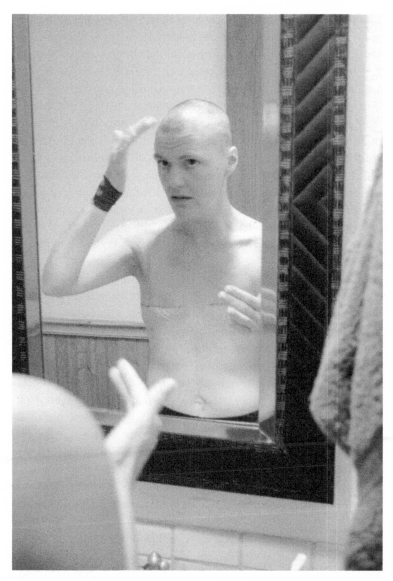

Amy S. Blackburn, *Torso in the Mirror.* © Amy S. Blackburn.

Blackburn also documents Ogden's hair loss and her quest for the right prosthesis. In one photograph viewers witness the haircut that chemo necessitates and Cynthia's wistful expression as blond curls fall to the floor; a subsequent image depicts her mother's impassive expression as she shaves her daughter's head. Another photograph, *Torso in the Mirror*, shows Cynthia looking in a bathroom mirror, examining her bald head with clinical detachment, her de-breasted chest visible in the mirror's reflection (51). Subsequent photos and Blackburn's narrative highlight Cynthia's struggle to achieve full range of motion in her shoulder and her confrontations with nausea, dehydration, blood transfusion, and memory loss—debilitating cycles for both patient and caregiver. Such indexical photographs contain ontological significance along with referential force: as Ulrich Baer notes, "the medium of photography always raises the question of the relationship between seeing and knowing" (1).[14]

Despite its powerful photographs and thoughtful narrative, *Caring for Cynthia* at times employs a triumphant discourse that may risk disavowing the dead. This discursive maneuver occurs primarily in Blackburn's preface, where she praises Cynthia's "will to survive," and in the afterword, where the photographer asserts that a year after surgery, "Cynthia is a breast cancer survivor. . . . She's unstoppable in achieving the goals that she sets for herself" (82). Although Blackburn includes photos of Cynthia's participation in a race sponsored by Susan G. Komen for the Cure and explains that this event honored the living and "memorialize[d] those who had not survived," the textual use of survivor discourse implies that survival is willed and praiseworthy, even regal. One unsettling photograph presents Cynthia looking pensively at the camera and wearing a tiara; in the accompanying narrative Blackburn calls Cynthia "a queen of endurance" (62). A less exotic but equally triumphant photo of a white bra hanging on a chain-link fence conveys a similar message: inscribed in blue magic marker on the right cup is "You can beat this" (80–81). Like the emphasis on victory in Myers's collection and on heroism in Nikpay's, the focus on triumph in *Caring for Cynthia* could alienate reader-viewers whose loved ones have died of breast cancer or who themselves are facing death. At its best, however, Blackburn's photo-documentary presents with sensitivity and compassion the breast cancer experiences of patient and care provider.

Memorial Discourses in *Knowing Stephanie*

Knowing Stephanie is the only photographic collection under consideration that is not only collaborative but coauthored. Stephanie Byram, its breast cancer subject, and Charlee Brodsky, her photographer, enjoyed a working relationship whose every aspect was mutually determined, from deciding what to photograph to correlating words and images to curating gallery exhibitions and developing websites.[15] Establishing coauthorship is important because, as Brodsky notes in her preface, Byram died two years before the book was published; hence this collection has an elegiac dimension. As Susan Sontag has argued, "all photographs are *memento mori*" in their representation of "lives hurtling toward their own destruction"; mortality gives life meaning, and any photograph documents the living while reinforcing the inevitability of death (*On Photography*, 3–4). Yet some photographs gesture more poignantly toward their subjects' mortality than others, and the images in *Knowing Stephanie* accrue power through the reader-viewer's awareness of the death of Byram, whose images portray a vibrant presence.

The fact that *Knowing Stephanie* was coauthored might also reassure reader-viewers that Stephanie gave this narrative her informed consent, since coauthorship is arguably one way of determining ethical efficacy. As Couser explains in *Vulnerable Subjects*, intimate biographical representations of subjects whose trust might easily be violated raise complex questions.

> Under what circumstances do life writers have ethical obligations to those they portray? More specifically, how does a cooperative relationship between subject and writer, such as authorization, affect the ethics of the project? . . . If life writing entails potential harms, such as violation of privacy, are they, can they, be offset by countervailing benefits? What good does life writing do, and whose interests does it finally serve—the subjects', the writers', or the readers'? (10)

Couser's questions help reader-viewers assess Byram and Brodsky's photo-documentary as ethical, given Byram's role as cocreator and adjudicator of her imagetext. Still, it is instructive to consider images that do *not* appear in *Knowing Stephanie*: photographs of Byram dying or deceased. Brodsky explains in her preface why she did not photograph Stephanie during her final days, "fragile, slight, recumbent" yet "a riveting presence."

> While looking at her, I saw many pictures and compositions. Many arrangements of her features through my camera's viewfinder would have been intensely melancholy and moving photographs. . . . But I never thought of bringing out my camera. Stephanie and I had always decided together when, where, and how to make our photographs—but while she was dying, she could not let me know what she wanted. Stephanie had been my subject, but she was also my collaborator. In this, our last experience together, I took her silence to be an invitation to leave my camera aside and to be present with her. I'm glad that there wasn't a camera between us. (Preface)

Brodsky honors discretion over revelation, unmediated closeness over camera-generated distance—and, arguably, ethics over aesthetics, since the vulnerable subject could not articulate her wishes. Yet vexed considerations of informed consent are rarely simple, as Brodsky acknowledges: "I don't know if Stephanie would have wanted me to photograph her that day. I made the decision not to on my own" (preface). From that moment forward the photo-documentary became a project of autothanatography and memorialization.[16]

Knowing Stephanie consists of eight sections whose titles convey its primary themes. "Diagnosis" depicts Byram's confrontation at thirty with a highly aggressive breast cancer, her subsequent bilateral mastectomy, and her frightening prognosis: "*The doctors gave me a 50 percent chance of surviving five years and a 40 percent chance of surviving ten years*" (12). Stephanie's narrative, however, emphasizes her subjectivity as well as her disease: "*This is me. This image tells a lot about me, but what it doesn't say is that I've had cancer*" (12). Here Byram authorizes the initial photographic image of her face; only later does she reveal her breastless chest, acknowledging in her commentary a sense of bodily betrayal: "*My body . . . could no longer be trusted, especially since I had treated it so well, with a nutritious diet and regular exercise. . . . I was no longer whole*" (20). This stark self-assessment is represented visually through a collage of Byram's body in pieces as the photographic subject lies prone, eyes tightly shut as if to avoid confronting her fragmentation. Yet her grief over what

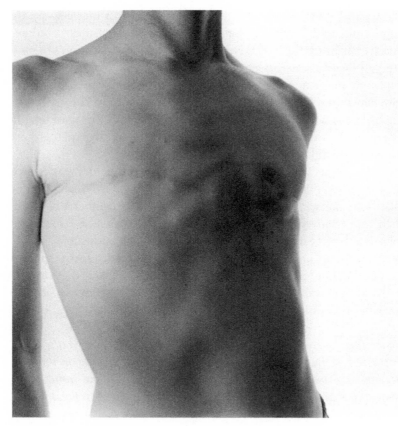

Charlee Brodsky, *Venus*. Courtesy of the artist.

she perceives as lost—"*Womanhood / Sexuality / Motherhood*"—is eventually transformed into an appreciation of who she is becoming. The catalyst for this ontological transformation, a photograph of Byram's post-mastectomy chest that Brodsky entitles *Venus*, reframes disfigurement as beauty, the fractured self as its own aesthetic: "*Like a Michelangelo sculpture with the arms knocked off, I now see my torso as a work of art. Although I'm missing some pieces, I no longer feel disfigured. This image was a turning point for me*" (26). The photograph's lighting draws attention to the taut musculature of Stephanie's chest, while its framing moves the viewer's eye both vertically, from the subject's strong shoulder to her narrow waist, and horizontally, from the smooth mastectomy scar on the right to its symmetrical counterpart on the left. "Venus caused a stir wherever it went," explains Jennifer Matesa in the biographical profile of Byram that concludes this collection; "survivors of mastectomy, on seeing Venus, told Stephanie that they never imagined they could see themselves as beautiful" (122). For some viewers the exhibition of *Venus* offered a powerful mirror; as Byram explains, "One woman, who also had bilateral mastectomies, had never seen another body like hers" (122). As Brodsky notes, Byram herself found in *Venus* not only a breast cancer aesthetic but also a source of rejuvenation: "Because of this photograph, I believe Stephanie was able to visualize herself differently and therefore was able to live differently" (11).

Subsequent sections of *Knowing Stephanie* document Byram's process of reconstructing her private and public selves. In "Searching for Balance" she narrates explicitly her efforts to "piece together a new self, unified and wonderfully alive" and to reclaim her sexuality. Two photographs that depict Stephanie embracing a male lover, both subjects nude from the waist up, are accompanied by a forthright claim and a troubled question: "Without breasts, my sexuality unalterably changed. As an unmarried woman, would men still be attracted to me?" Yet Byram goes on to trace her process of self-acceptance.

> *Later I discovered that I still lusted after the same men who were attractive to me before my diagnosis. Unexpectedly acting on those feelings, I experienced an awakening that liberated me from the stereotypes and fears of owning a "mutilated" body. My flat torso simply didn't matter; the chemistry and the intense passion were the same.* (39)

Unlike *Winged Victory,* in which romantic love is presented as transcendent, *Knowing Stephanie* foregrounds its subject's shifting awareness of the force of her eroticism. In addition, Byram refutes the notion that a sexual partner is necessary for a post-mastectomy woman, although having one can be pleasurable. "*A woman doesn't need a man,*" reads the narrative that accompanies two additional photographs of Stephanie and her male companion, "*but having you is awfully nice. Ours is a relationship of tenderness, trust, intimacy, and relaxed togetherness, signs of security in our familiarity*" (70). One untitled rearview photograph depicts the upper body of Stephanie, bald and clad in a tank top, beside a shirtless male companion whose arm is comfortably thrown around her shoulder. Brodsky has acknowledged this untitled image as one of her favorites from the collection: "For me, it's about human closeness, with

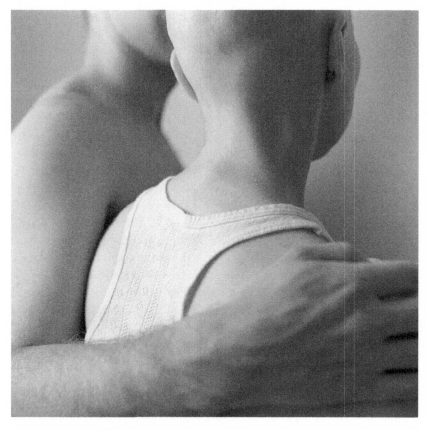

Charlee Brodsky, *Untitled.* Courtesy of the artist.

skin touching skin."[17] *Knowing Stephanie* clearly gestures toward feminism in its celebration of women's erotic desire and its honoring of the power of human touch.

Byram and Brodsky's commitment to cancer activism is the subject of "Finding My Place," which highlights Stephanie's decision to run in thirty of the Komen Foundation's annual Races for the Cure. Several photographs present her in shorts and T-shirt looking gleeful: "*My goals are to raise one hundred thousand dollars for breast cancer research and to raise awareness of breast cancer*" (44). Also noteworthy from a feminist perspective are Byram's verbal challenge to patriarchal society's breast fetish—"'*Clothes don't make a man.' And breasts don't make a woman*"—and her refusal to consider reconstruction (55). As Matesa notes, "Choosing not to reconstruct her breasts was perhaps the pivotal decision Stephanie made during her experience with cancer" because "it is clear from her writings that Stephanie perceived a great deal of pressure from the medical community and the culture at large to rebuild the body parts that had been taken by cancer" (114). As Byram explains in her commentary, this decision was nonnegotiable: "Breast reconstruction never seemed like the right choice to me. . . . The more I learned about it, the more it turned me off. . . . If women want to have reconstruction, if they want to have implants, if they want to wear prostheses, great. But I think they should be given some information about not having reconstruction, as well" (114, 116). Like Audre Lorde in *The Cancer Journals,* Byram considers her decision against reconstruction not only principled but necessary for her well-being: "*If I reconstruct my body, I will not be able to reconstruct my life*" (117). In addition, she claims hairlessness and breastlessness as beautiful; one photograph of her bald head is accompanied by an impassioned defense of nonconformity: "*Why is it that I never see anyone without hair? Why is it that my doctor insisted that I would want to 'reconstruct' my breasts? Is it so important to hide our appearances, to hide our cancers? Why should I feel ashamed? Is it so important to conform, to avert the stares and whispers?*" (86). In such passages Byram critiques breast cancer cultural hegemony and dissects the politics of appearance.

An unflinching emphasis on multiple recurrences distinguishes this photo-documentary from the other visual narratives under consideration here, as reader-viewers witness Stephanie's confrontation with lymphatic tumors two years after her diagnosis, with bone, liver, and brain metastases in the years to follow. The haunting photograph that Byram and Brodsky chose to inaugurate this section of the narrative, entitled *Recurrence,* was taken on Stephanie's thirty-second birthday shortly after cancer had returned in her left armpit; in it she strolls through a barren forest in a trench coat, bald and visible only from behind. Stephanie knew the seriousness of this development, Brodsky explains in the narrative; for this reason the photograph resembled for both photographer and subject "a World War II image. Very grim and ominous, with a desolate landscape" (121). For Matesa, however, this image presents Byram "treading a path. Her head is up; she is stepping over the obstacles in her way; she is wearing protective clothing; she is holding onto a tree for support; she is going somewhere. She is moving into the unfamiliar" (121).

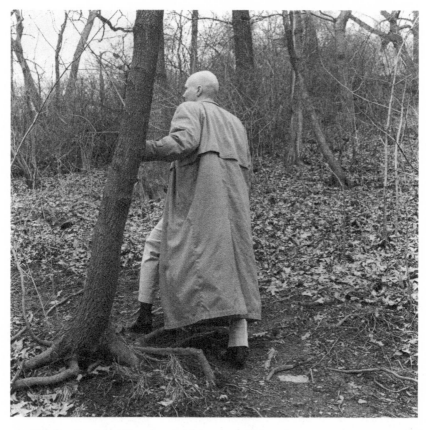

Charlee Brodsky, *Recurrence*. Courtesy of the artist.

Stephanie exudes a quiet strength in this photograph and in other final portraits, a quality evident in the accompanying narratives: "*Struggling for a sense of balance, I now live with an emotional intensity, full of spirit and hope*" (96). This discourse of hope differs from that of *Heroines,* for Stephanie acknowledges without self-pity that she will soon die of her disease; until then, however, she is determined to live. Toward the end of *Knowing Stephanie* reader-viewers witness Byram in calm repose, arm thrown casually over her bald head as she sleeps. This intimate photograph seizes power through its capacity, in Barthes's words, to convey "at the same time 'this will be' and 'this has been' . . . an anterior future of which death is the stake" (96). It signals the irreplaceable loss of Stephanie that is to come.

Transformational Encounters with Breast
Cancer Photographs

How might readers and viewers best assess the aesthetic, documentary,
and ethical dimensions of postmillennial breast cancer photo-narratives?
What forms of spectatorial engagement do visual and verbal representations of women's post-operative, scarred, and recovering or dying bodies
invite? As Timothy Dow Adams points out in *Life Writing/Light Writing*,
in autobiography, photographic image and text function as interactive
and mutually reflective; they complement rather than supplement one
another. Although conventional autobiographical theory has sometimes
considered photographs merely as visual tools corroborating a written
text, Adams rightly counters that "both media are highly self-conscious,
and combining them may intensify rather than reduce the complexity
and ambiguity of each taken separately" (xx). Such is the case in the
breast cancer photo-narratives examined in this chapter.

Griselda Pollock has argued persuasively that photographic narratives that inscribe traumatic occurrences have the capacity to lead viewers toward "transformational encounters that can be processed without
[the] usual risks of Orphic voyeurism, inured familiarity, or sublime pa-
thos" ("Dying, Seeing, Feeling," 231). Such encounters are by no means
guaranteed, for "as a created borderspace, art is neither pure content nor
image nor mere expression. It creates an *occasion* for subjectivity to be
affected along strings or cords that run through an object or a process
of creation" (231). For visually and emotionally empathic encounters to
occur, photographs of women suffering or recovering from breast cancer must "bring into view both the ethical, the relationship or openness
to the Other, and the aesthetic, as an instance of a noncognitive trans-
ferential possibility of changing the inner world of another" (231). One
strategy for approaching breast cancer photographs transferentially involves what Kaja Silverman has termed "productive looking": "The ethical becomes operative not at the moment when unconscious desire and
phobias assume possession of our look, but in a subsequent moment,
when we take stock of what we have just 'seen' and attempt . . . to look
again, differently" (173). Unlike spectatorial gazes in which a subject objectifies an Other through attempts at visual mastery, productive looking
requires active identification with whoever is beheld, as well as vigilant
self-monitoring, which Silverman describes as "a constant, conscious

reworking of the terms under which we unconsciously look at the objects that people our visual landscape" (184). If we as reader-viewers engage in productive looking and openly encounter photographic images of women traumatized by breast cancer, our inner and intersubjective landscapes can be transformed.

6 | Cancer Narratives and an Ethics of Commemoration
Susan Sontag, Annie Leibovitz, and David Rieff

Susan Sontag's cultural critique of cancer stigmatization in *Illness as Metaphor* (1977) and her theoretical musings in *On Photography* (1977) and *Regarding the Pain of Others* (2003) offer rich insights through which to analyze photographic and literary representations of Sontag's own experience with cancer by Annie Leibovitz (her lover) in *A Photographer's Life, 1990–2005* and David Rieff (Sontag's son) in his 2008 memoir, *Swimming in a Sea of Death*. My analysis in this chapter raises ethical as well as aesthetic issues important to postmillennial understandings of cancer as a sociopolitical construct and an individual disease, and of the ways that cancer patients and their ill, medicalized, suffering, and dying bodies have been and might justly be represented in literature and art. I hope ultimately to shed light on debates regarding appropriate versus appropriative depictions of people with cancer and to raise questions from a feminist perspective that might help readers consider what constitutes an ethics of commemoration.

In *Illness as Metaphor* Sontag examines the traumatic and transformational power of life-threatening diseases, which force the humans who contract them to face "the night side of life," relinquishing their place in "the kingdom of the well" for "a more onerous citizenship in that other place" (1). Specifically, she compares the nineteenth-century quest to eliminate tuberculosis with twentieth-century efforts to eradicate cancer and discusses the ways in which both diseases are "spectacularly, and similarly, encumbered by the trappings of metaphor" (5). Tuberculosis and cancer have long evoked terror and dread, she explains; physicians have described these diseases as *consuming, corrupting, insidious,* while the culture at large has deemed them *unspeakable, monstrous.* For cancer patients, portrayed in life and in art as "humiliated by fear and agony," such language may exacerbate suffering and self-blame; certainly "the people who have the real disease are hardly helped by hearing their disease's name constantly being dropped as the epitome of evil" (80). If cancer can be stripped of negative metaphors and "de-mythicized," Sontag argues, ill people can avoid stigmatization and address cancer on their own terms (86–87).[1]

Illness as Metaphor has served for more than thirty years as an incisive text for interrogating the dehumanization that cancer patients have experienced at the hands of some medical practitioners and in the cultural imagination. Although she did not acknowledge it until years later, Sontag wrote this book shortly after her own treatment, at forty-two, for stage-four metastatic breast cancer, which she survived for over twenty years through a combination of radical mastectomy, aggressive chemotherapy, and then-experimental immunotherapy pioneered by French physician Lucien Israël. She later spoke proudly of "confounding my doctors' pessimism" (Rieff, 25). In 1998 Sontag was treated for a rare type of uterine cancer, for which she also underwent successful chemotherapy, and early in 2004 she was diagnosed with myelodysplastic syndrome (MDS), a malignant blood cancer probably caused by her previous chemotherapies. In December 2004, after an unsuccessful bone marrow transplant, Sontag died of MDS. Although she published no autobiographical accounts of her cancer experience, Leibovitz's photographic narrative and Rieff's "son's memoir" have provoked controversy among viewers, readers, and reviewers over the tensions between humiliation and memorialization, between voyeurism and empathy: tensions that Sontag herself probed in *On Photography*, which explores the relationship of photographic representation to morality and knowledge, and in *Regarding the Pain of Others*, which examines the effects on viewers of horrific images of war, violence, and human suffering.[2] Among the topics these texts invite readers to explore are patients' rights issues of who has the authority to represent another person's experience of cancer and what parameters should exist with regard to such representation, as well as theoretical issues of the reader-viewer's position via a potentially exploitative gaze/look/stare. Sontag's work, Leibovitz's photographs, and Rieff's memoir also evoke ongoing debates in photographic theory regarding documentary versus aesthetically driven art photography, cultural issues of death denial and representations of trauma in contemporary society, and feminist issues of female subjectivity, lesbian visibility, and reciprocal witness among writer or photographer, her or his subject, and audience.

Leibovitz's *A Photographer's Life*, both the 2006 book and the traveling exhibition housed from October 2008 to February 2009 at the National

Portrait Gallery in London and more recently shown in Berlin, Madrid, and Vienna, consists of large, airbrushed, highly stylized, lushly colored photos of celebrities that have earned her the designation "American master" and a series of mostly small, informal black-and-white photos of her parents, children, siblings, friends, and lover (Somerstein, np).[3] Of the more than 300 images contained in the book, which Leibovitz calls "a memoir in photographs," two-thirds are personal, and approximately a hundred of these depict Sontag (Guthmann, np). In many photos she appears as a traveler reflecting upon an exotic landscape, an artist at work either writing or directing theater, a woman engaged in conversation with friends or gazing at her lover's newborn child, or a domestic partner relaxing in a shared and sometimes eroticized space, most often bath or bed. The remaining photos present Sontag hospitalized and hooked up to machines, receiving chemo at home, recovering from a bone marrow transplant, dying—and finally dead, elegantly dressed for burial. Leibovitz has acknowledged that these photos are "tough" and "contentious" but explains that "every single image that one would have a possible problem with or have concerns about, I had them too. . . . And I made the decision in the long run that the strength of the book needed these pictures, and the fact that it came out of a moment of grief gave the work dignity" (Scott, np).

In her introduction to *A Photographer's Life* Leibovitz claims that selecting the cancer photographs for inclusion was an important part of her grieving process, that she edited the book "with [Sontag] in mind, as if she were standing behind me, saying what she would like to see in it" and that, if alive, Sontag "would champion the work" (np). Part of the ethical ambiguity of these images rests in Leibovitz's silence as to whether she had Sontag's permission to take and to publish such intimate, sometimes graphic photographs; the standard code of ethics in public photography requires photographers to acquire their subject's consent for access but not necessarily for future use.[4] In a 2006 interview Leibovitz equivocates with regard to publication rights: "I think Susan would be really proud of those pictures—but she's dead. Now if she were alive, she would not want them published. It's really a difference. It's really strange." Ultimately, however, Leibovitz concludes that she has "been through everything mentally and emotionally, and I'm very comfortable with them" (McGuigan, np).[5] Her ethical gauges, therefore, become the presumed approval of the deceased photographic subject and her own good intentions as artist and mourner.

Complicating any scholarly analysis of Leibovitz's photographic representation of Sontag's cancers is the position that her son, David Rieff, assumes in his narrative of his mother's final year, *Swimming in a Sea of Death.* There Rieff reveals in painful detail Sontag's struggle with MDS in all its desperation, courage, banality, and poignancy; he chronicles as well as his uncertainty as to whether he should have supported her decision "to do everything she could to save her life," his sense of "psychological intubation" during her various hospitalizations, and his survivors' guilt (101, 118). Despite the fact that his mother and Leibovitz were lovers for fifteen years, Rieff makes only two references to the photographer in his memoir, the first of which describes her as Sontag's "on-again, off-again companion of many years"—a description, as one British reviewer notes, that makes Leibovitz "sound like an unsatisfactory family retainer" (Rieff, 66; Mars-Jones, np). The second and more substantial reference raises the issue of ethical commemoration.

> If there really were some benevolent god or world spirit inclined to meddle in the affairs of human beings, or at least to shelter them from what they most feared, my mother would not have died slowly and painfully from MDS but suddenly from a massive heart attack—the death that all of us who, like my mother (and like me), are crippled by the fear of extinction must yearn for. Sometimes I have actually visualized it. . . . She would not have had the time to mourn herself and to become physically unrecognizable at the end even to herself, let alone humiliated posthumously by being "memorialized" that way in those carnival images of celebrity death taken by Annie Leibovitz. (149–50)

This passage merits close examination not only because of Rieff's rage and grief but also for the light it sheds on the complexities of envisioning appropriate forms of memorialization. The sentence "I have actually visualized it" establishes the son's self-authorizing gesture to create counterimages different from those that Leibovitz's book and exhibition, and for that matter his own memory, offer—an imaginative seizure of what Roland Barthes has termed a "*camera lucida*" to replace the shadowy "*camera obscura*" whose optic images distort (80). Rieff's use of the subjunctive clause "She would not have had the time . . ." reinforces his recurring claims that his dying mother spent months despairing over her future, torn between hope that she could yet achieve her latest goals as a writer and fear that this third cancer would prove fatal. The infinitive phrase "to mourn herself" provides a self-reflexive alternative to conventional idioms of lamenting one's decline, illness, or incipient death (for what does it mean, finally, to mourn one's *self*?). And the phrase "to become physically unrecognizable at the end even to herself" raises questions about who is looking—who has the right to look—at pictures of a dying cancer patient, what kind of introspective or external gaze is acceptable, and what physical and psychological damage to patient and loved ones is exacted by a disease that leaves a human being alienated from her own image in the mirror and renders a maternal body abject before her tormented son.

The final sentences of Rieff's bitter passage raise issues that Sontag explores in *Illness as Metaphor* and *On Photography* regarding cancer as a disease too often seen as shameful, photography as both an elegiac art ("all photographs are *memento mori*") and an intrusive one, and the nature and morality of spectatorship (Sontag, *On Photography*, 15). "In teaching us a new visual code," Sontag claims, "photographs alter and enlarge our notions of what is worth looking at and what we have a right to observe. They are a grammar and, even more importantly, an ethics of seeing" (*On Photography*, 3). Rieff's phrase "humiliated posthumously" references what his mother refers to as ethical seeing; at first glance his phrase seems oxymoronic, since surely one must be alive to experience humiliation, yet it lambastes Leibovitz for allegedly violating Sontag's privacy by making a spectacle of her dying and dead body. Rieff's attribution of humiliation to Sontag seems ironic, given her insistence in *Illness as Metaphor* that cancer should be viewed as a disease, not a stigma. Nonetheless, the son's condemnation of what he considers his mother's posthumous shaming further raises questions regarding the power of a camera to wound/distort or, conversely, to offer a cruelly indexical representation rather than a generously iconic one. Rieff's phrase "'memorialized' that way," with the verb placed in angrily dismissive quotation marks, again asks readers implicitly to consider what constitutes an acceptable memorial representation ("that way" referring back to the issue of recognition). And the phrase "those carnival images of celebrity death" recalls both Sylvia Plath's horror and titillation at the "peanut crunching crowd" who mock a suicidal woman in "Lady Lazarus" and Mikhail Bakhtin's analysis of the power of carnival to attract voyeuristic audiences more interested in jeering "flawed" embodiment and enjoying dehumanizing spectacle than in celebrating creative performance or human difference (Plath, 14–17; Bakhtin, 154). In this final phrase Rieff condemns Leibovitz as a commercial photographer who exploits the vulnerable Sontag via the camera's diminishing lens.

Empathy and Accountability in Leibovitz's
Illness Photographs

How might viewers determine what constitutes an ethical photographic representation of another person's suffering and death from cancer and an empathic rather than a voyeuristic response to such photographs, using Leibovitz's images and Rieff's critique as a case study? Let us turn now to eight images/image sequences of Sontag from *A Photographer's Life* and apply Sontag's photographic theory to consider this question. The first Leibovitz photograph, identified as *Residencia Santo Spirito, Milan, 1991,* is prominently located three pages after the book's dedication page; it features Sontag lying on a bed that functions as a writer's desk, notes and papers strewn about, a typewriter on a table to the left. The subject gazes directly at the photographer/camera with gentle, loving eyes and a slight aura of weariness, perhaps at the endless and formidable task of writing. Sontag's elegant fingers and outstretched hands are featured, as is her body's delicate curve and her famous long, dark hair with its dramatic white streak fanned out against the pillow. There is no sign of illness, and consent to photograph is evident in the reciprocal gaze of photographer and subject, with which the viewer can comfortably engage and from which draw aesthetic pleasure.

The second photograph, a series labeled *My Apartment in London Terrace, West 23rd Street, New York, 1992,* juxtaposes four frames of Sontag, nude, relaxing in her lover's bathtub, her hand covering her post-surgical left breast. Sontag's face is visible only in the upper left frame, which also reveals traces of her mastectomy scar, barely covered by her left arm. What Barthes calls the *punctum* of a moving photograph—that prick or shock of recognition that evokes identification or compassion or perhaps dread—occurs for me via the pouches under the subject's arm that appear in the other three frames, an image that indicates as well the photograph's *studium*—the cultural and historical context that helps one interpret it—by signifying the ravages of breast cancer surgery when the patient has lymph node involvement (27–28). Leibovitz's representation of Sontag's body, her mastectomy scar, her puckered underarm skin, and (in three frames) her torso only (sans face) may unsettle the viewer, who feels she or he has stumbled onto a private scene. As Marianne Hirsch asks in *Family Frames*, "What happens when a [closed, familial] circle is enlarged to include other viewers and readers? . . . What are the ethics, what are the politics, of this 'exposure,' this public reading of images that generate their meanings in the private realm?" (107). Affiliation or alienation can result, Hirsch posits, or a vexed combination that leaves viewers feeling ambivalent or even complicit in an act of violation. In this case, however, because Sontag is fully conscious and presumably aware that the photos are being taken, neither violation nor permission is an issue, though consent to publish might be. Since Leibovitz has assured viewers, however, that taking intimate pictures is both a privilege and a responsibility to which she has tried to be accountable, and since the photos of Sontag's scars are part of a culturally familiar body of U.S. mastectomy photographs displayed from the 1970s to the present, this photographic sequence of Sontag seems unlikely to strike most viewers as exploitative.[6]

The next three photographic sequences, taken during and shortly after Sontag's 1998 treatment for uterine cancer, depict what Leibovitz considers a documentary collaboration between the two women. In the first set of images, frames five through eight from a series captioned *Mt. Sinai Hospital, New York, July 1998,* Sontag is lying in a hospital bed, undressed perhaps for a bath, covered by a towel and clutching a pillow. In the top two frames her melancholy gaze is directed at neither camera nor photographer, but she seems calm; in the lower left frame, however, she looks anxious, hand clutching the bed frame as the nurse probes or cleans her partially exposed buttocks. The lower right frame restores the patient's agency, since the nurse and she are conversing; Sontag is now clothed in a hospital gown and seems to lie in bed comfortably, left arm and legs outstretched. A related pair of images from August 1998, entitled *Susan Receiving Chemotherapy, and, above, with Ben Yeoman at 24th Street, August 1998,* emphasizes Sontag's restoration. In the top frame she has returned home and is back at work, manuscript and assistant at hand. In the bottom frame viewers witness the aftereffects of her cancer in the form of ongoing chemotherapy via port, administered by a visiting nurse. Most riveting is Sontag's range of expressions: intense engagement with her manuscript, an accepting half-smile for the nurse. A second dyad, entitled *Bertilda Garcia Cutting Susan's Hair, West 24th Street, August 1998,* is juxtaposed with the chemotherapy photographs and portrays

Sontag receiving a radical haircut necessitated presumably by the hair loss expected to accompany chemo. In the top frame she gazes grimly at the camera as Garcia trims her white streak; the bottom frame offers a mirror reflection of Sontag's sober confrontation with her new bobbed visage. To interpret these photographic sequences viewers can turn again to Barthes's *studium,* for Sontag's experience offers a cultural narrative familiar to most cancer patients, who after hospitalization must balance return to work with ongoing chemo and likely baldness—the latter causing a significant strain for women in general and perhaps for Sontag in particular, given that beautiful hair signifies hegemonic femininity and that Sontag's celebrity rested on her striking looks as well as her writing.

The four-frame strategy used often by Leibovitz provides her photographic sequences with narrative depth and flow. As she explains in *A Photographer's Life,* she stumbled upon this technique when selecting photos for the book after the deaths of both Sontag and Leibovitz's father, who died six weeks later and whose decline she also chronicled. She grouped photos at first for convenience but soon realized that "the result was unexpectedly powerful. The pictures created portraits that were like little films. It wasn't a single moment. It was a flow of images, which is more like life" (np). The photographs that make up this 1998 "film" of Sontag hospitalized, then back at home offer a poignant cancer narrative in images—a narrative in which cancer survivor, photographer, and viewer are reciprocally involved. All of the images of Sontag examined thus far seem ethically unambiguous in that access appears freely granted and the subject is an active participant. Moreover, these images reassure viewers in their "restitutive" movement (Arthur Frank's term) from diagnosis to treatment to healing—the dominant cancer narrative endorsed by the American Cancer Society, whose discourse strives, as Sandra Gilbert has noted, to associate cancer not with death but with recovery (Frank, 135–37; Gilbert, 105–6).

The last three photographic sequences encode trauma and death; they have thus evoked protest, not only from Rieff but also from reviewers such as Sarah Karnasiewicz, who criticizes Liebovitz's "reckless candor" and "unseemly striving," and David Thomson, who calls them "voyeuristic shots of death's moment, which is the most individualized, the most private, moment of all." Indeed, Thomson further claims that "without consent, they seem to me unpublishable, and much more distressing than the photographer knows" (Karnasiewicz, np; Thomson, np). Leibovitz *does* know, however: she admits in *A Photographer's Life* that these photos are "harrowing" and that initially she did not want to "be there as a photographer" at Sontag's bedside; rather, "I just wanted to be there." Yet once she realized that Sontag was dying, she felt both a sense of urgency and a desire to pay homage to their earlier collaboration: "I forced myself to take pictures of Susan's last days. Perhaps the pictures completed the work she and I had begun together when she was sick in 1998. I didn't analyze it then. I just knew I had to do it" (np). Hence Leibovitz claims both artistic license and a history of intimacy to justify this project.

The three-frame sequence entitled *University of Washington Medical Center, Seattle, Washington, November 2004*, taken just after her bone marrow transplant, displays a hospitalized, unconscious woman no longer visually identifiable as Susan Sontag. Her sweeping streaked hair has been replaced by a wispy white cap, her face and body are swollen, her arms and legs are bruised, and she is connected to a maze of wires. In the top two frames she lies on her back, mouth open as if she might be having trouble breathing; in the lower frame she rests on her right side, a tube extending from her bandaged left leg. A related photograph, *Leaving Seattle, November 15, 2004*, shows Sontag unconscious and lying on a stretcher poised on the tarmac beside the private airplane that would convey her from Seattle home to New York to die a few weeks later. Two airline personnel work to adjust the stretcher, seemingly determining how best to load it for medical evacuation. A final photograph, *New York, December 29, 2004*, which presents Sontag's embalmed corpse lying on a funeral home table, her face serene, recalls a nineteenth-century tableau of *memento mori*.[7] This image jolts most twenty-first-century viewers, for as cultural critics from Julia Kristeva to Elisabeth Bronfen have noted, the modern fear of death is so pronounced that Western cultures have made the human corpse taboo, the ultimate signifier of abjection. The dead Sontag is dressed in clothing that Leibovitz meticulously selected as a means of commemorating a vibrant life of art and travel.

> After she died, I chose the clothes she would be buried in and took them to Frank Campbell's funeral home myself. The dress is one we found in Milan. It's an homage to Fortuny, made the way he made them, with pleated material. . . . Susan had been sick on and off for several years, in the hospital for months. It's humiliating. You lose yourself. And she loved to dress up. I brought scarves we had bought in Venice and a black velvet Yeohlee coat that she

wore to the theater. I was in a trance when I took the pictures of her lying there. (np)

In this passage Leibovitz agrees with Rieff that cancer humiliated Sontag by robbing her of agency and dignity, yet she clearly intends this depiction of her stilled lover, luminous and ritually dressed in beautiful clothing, as a photographic memorialization that works *against* humiliation by restoring Sontag's elegance and their shared history. Sartorial restitution, however, does not necessarily restore Sontag's privacy and dignity, or so Rieff has argued in decrying both the Washington Medical Center and the funeral home photographs as "carnival images of celebrity death." Still, Rieff's accusation may be countered by the fact that Leibovitz also chronicles her father's decline and death from cancer in *A Photographer's Life,* thereby blurring the boundary between private and public commemoration.

Sontag's theories from *Regarding the Pain of Others* offer insight into trauma photographs that can help us evaluate the ethical dimensions of these photos of her own death from cancer, although it is important to note that she developed these theories in response to modern representations of war and genocide, from the Holocaust to Bosnia to Abu Ghraib, not to representations of death from disease. Nonetheless, she accurately notes that "the iconography of suffering has a long pedigree. The sufferings most often deemed worthy of representation are those understood to be the product of wrath, divine or human. (Suffering from natural causes, such as illness or childbirth, is scantily represented in the history of art . . .)" (40). The dangers of trauma photographs, once rare, but ubiquitous and thus potentially anesthetizing in twenty-first-century U.S. society, include both the exploitation of subjects captured without their knowledge at times of violence and the "exploitation of [viewer] sentiment (pity, compassion, indignation)" (80).[8] Sontag raises questions about trauma photos applicable to any consideration of Leibovitz's photos of her: "What is the point of exhibiting these pictures? To awaken indignation? To make us feel 'bad'; that is, to appall and sadden? To help us mourn? . . . Are we the better for seeing these images?" (91–92). Leibovitz has explained why she took illness photos of Sontag and what they meant to her but has addressed only obliquely the question of why private images should be made public: "People have said that it's important to publish them because so much is masked for us about what the end really is" (McGuigan, np). This argument has merit: in a culture obsessed with death denial, where corpses are hidden away in funeral homes until embalming or cremation rather than washed, dressed, and displayed at home for family and friends to mourn, as was done in earlier centuries in America and is still done in many parts of the world, it seems important that the veil be removed.[9] Unlike our culture's familiar and horrific photos of the human casualties of war and atrocities, photos of ill people suffering are relatively rare, yet they too deserve representation.

Mourning and Melancholia in Rieff's Son's Memoir

While photographic representations of the dying strike some viewers as ethically suspect, especially when the subjects have not granted explicit permission, written texts in which sons reckon with their mothers' deaths generally receive a positive cultural reception, as witnessed by critical praise for such diverse works as Barthes's *Camera Lucida,* cartoonist Brian Fies's graphic memoir *Mom's Cancer,* and Rieff's memoir of Sontag's final months. Intriguingly, ethical considerations of access, consent, taste, and decency do not emerge in most reviews of Rieff's book, perhaps because U.S. readers and reviewers take for granted a journalist-son's right to chronicle his famous mother's demise—indeed, it is seen as a sign of filial love—whereas, due perhaps to homophobia and/or misogyny, some condemn a lesbian photographer's documentation of her well-known lover's decline. Yet Rieff's memoir is as grimly revelatory as Leibovitz's photographs, as will become clear when we analyze the ways in which his text exposes raw and private aspects of Sontag's cancer experience. His memoir thus serves as a second case study for determining what constitutes an ethical narrative commemoration.

Early on Rieff explores his mother's declining ability to use words, a hallmark of her professional identity, when coping with her diagnosis of MDS, and her subsequent despair. When Sontag and Rieff visit her oncologist's office in January 2004 to learn the results of tests taken to investigate suspicious lesions, he explains, they receive the curt verdict that Sontag has a virulent, virtually untreatable blood cancer. After a long silence and a shocked question to the physician—"So what you're telling me . . . is that in fact there is nothing to be done. . . . Nothing I can do."—Sontag left the office with Rieff, remained silent during their drive home, and finally responded only, "Wow" (10–11). In the following weeks she summoned language only intermittently, "through the choking haze of her own panic": "Disoriented and despairing, she oscillated between a hyper-manic wakefulness and intensity and a bedraggled somnolence. When I would come to her apartment, I felt as if I could feel the ghosts of stillborn screams" (46). A writer famed for her brilliant use of words is thus "outed" by her son as having been rendered inarticulate by her cancer diagnosis.

Rieff further reveals that years earlier Sontag had responded with fear and depression to her breast cancer diagnosis, her Halsted mastectomy, and her subsequent chemotherapy—and responded in ways contrary to her anti-stigmatizing argument in *Illness as Metaphor*. Explaining that her unpublished journal entries from that period are "punctuated with the repeated notation: 'Cancer = death,'" he also documents her private use of military metaphors, to which she vehemently objects in her public writing. "One [doctor] pushes and pulls and pokes, admiring his handi-work, my vast scar," writes Sontag. "The other pumps me full of poison, to kill my disease but not me. . . . I feel like the Vietnam War. . . . My body is invasive, colonizing. They're using chemical weapons on me. I have to cheer" (Rieff, 28, 35). Rieff notes that Sontag laments repeatedly in her 1975 journals about "how diminished she feels": "'People speak of illness as deepening,' she writes. 'I don't feel deepened. I feel flattened. I've become opaque to myself.' But at the same time, she keeps asking herself how she can transform this feeling. Is there some way, she de-mands, that she can 'turn it into a liberation'?" (Rieff, 35). Despite Son-tag's attempts to wrest meaning from her initial cancer experience, Rieff concludes, "Reading her diaries after her death, I am overwhelmed not by the force of her will . . . but rather on the depth of her despair," which takes the form of a traditional mind-body split. "While I was busy zap-ping the world with my mind, my body fell down," wrote Sontag. "I've become afraid of my own imagination" (Rieff, 41). Rieff further claims that despite his mother's intellectual refutation of psychologist Wilhelm Reich's assertion that "sexual repression" caused cancer, she believed it on an emotional level: "'I feel my body has let me down,' she wrote. 'And my mind, too. For, somewhere, I believe the Reichian verdict. I'm re-sponsible for my cancer. I lived as a coward, repressing my desire, my rage'" (Rieff, 36). For generations of Sontag readers, many of them cancer patients inspired by her incisive critical insights in *Illness as Metaphor*, Rieff's exposure of Sontag's private assimilation of patient-blaming dis-courses that she publicly refuted reveals more than she—or we—might have wished.

Rieff goes on to assert his mother's belief in her own exceptional-ism and to present her as self-aggrandizing. "My mother came to being ill imbued with a profound sense of being the exception to every rule," he explains . . . "If she no longer could believe herself exempt from the humiliations of the flesh, there was a way in which she came to believe that she would indeed be the exception" (144, 146). After all, she had survived stage-four breast cancer by exerting her own fierce determina-tion; as Rieff notes, "she believed in her own will, and, grandiose though it may seem, in her own star. Such belief is easy to mock. But everything my mother accomplished, and she accomplished a lot, was undergirded by that belief" (29). When MDS struck, Sontag told her son, "'This time, for the first time in my life, I don't feel special.'" Musing later on this statement, Rieff suggests, "It was that sense of being special . . . that had allowed her to both get through her two previous cancers and, retrospec-tively at least, to view the fact of having survived the disease as somehow more than a statistical accident or the luck of the biological draw. . . . She *did* believe that she was 'special' in exactly the way so many artists do" (85–86). Rieff's narrative thus invests his mother with a narcissism that readers may accept or may object to as an oedipally driven form of judgment.

Rieff also reveals how much Sontag suffered from her final cancer, how adamantly she refused to discuss death, and how desperately she insisted that he reassure her with any "over-hyped stories" he could find online about miraculous instances of MDS survival. Amazed that his mother remained "unreconciled to mortality" even "after suffering so much pain—and God, what pain she suffered!" Rieff asserts that her final illness and invasive medical treatment "had stripped her both of physi-cal dignity and mental acuity" (13, 103). Although he longed to talk with her about dying, "I was not going to raise the subject unless she did. It was her death, not mine. And she did not raise it. To do so would have been to concede that she might die and what she wanted was survival, not extinction—survival on any terms" (17). Since Sontag employed a strategy that Rieff describes as "positive denial," her son felt obligated to fabricate good news: "What she wanted from me was an adamant re-fusal to accept that it was even *possible* that she might not survive. . . . In the morning, I might be visiting my mother in her hospital room and, though she might be covered in sores, incontinent, and half delirious, tell her at great and cheerful length about how much better she seemed to look/seem/be compared to the day before" (128–30). While Rieff understandably focuses his narrative on the toll this vexed strategy took on his own psyche, his graphic account provides as well a disturbing portrait of Sontag's wounded embodiment and psychological distress.[10]

Finally, Rieff probes his mother's response to her futile last surgery and the words she muttered in her final delirium. Discussing Sontag's treatment of last resort, her bone marrow transplant of November 2004, he provides a harrowing description of her physical transformation that might well accompany the Leibovitz photographs taken at University of Washington Medical Center to which Rieff vehemently objected.

> Bedridden in the aftermath of her bone marrow transplant, her muscles soon so flaccid and wasted that she was unable even to roll over unaided, her flesh increasingly ulcerated, and her mouth so cankered that she was often unable to swallow and sometimes unable even to speak, she dreamt (and spoke, when she could speak, that is) of what she could do when she got out of the hospital and once more took up the reins of her life. The future was everything. Living was everything. Getting back to work was everything. (104–5)

Despite her ongoing hope of recovery, which Rieff considered "irrational," Sontag declined over the next month and on the day before her death again wrestled with words, in and out of consciousness. "By then, she was not speaking to any of those around her except to ask to be turned in her bed, or given water, or to ask for the nurse. But she had been speaking a lot, in a low tone, and seemingly to herself, about her mother and about a great love of a much earlier period of her life, Joseph Brodsky" (162). Rieff's arguably sensationalizing revelation of his mother's delirious musings evokes readers' empathy at a dying woman's life review even as it risks awakening voyeuristic curiosity about Sontag's relationship with the dissident writer Brodsky, himself recently deceased. Her last words to her son, Rieff notes, were fragmented: "But after a pause, she said, 'I want to tell you . . . ' That was all she said. She gestured vaguely with one emaciated hand and then let it drop onto the coverlet" (162–3).

Like Leibovitz, Rieff remains silent as to whether he sought or attained Sontag's permission to publish details of her death. Neither does he speculate as to how his mother would respond were she alive to read his words. Like Leibovitz, who claims that she did not want to sit at Sontag's bedside as a photographer but wanted only to be there, Rieff explains in his memoir and in interviews that he took no notes during his mother's final illness because he wished to avoid the detached writer's "sliver of ice in the heart" and instead to be there only as a son (106).[11] And like Leibovitz, Rieff has acknowledged that his choice to represent publicly Sontag's cancer experience and his role in it emerged gradually as part of his grief work and his desire to pay homage to her.

"Encountering the Ethical as the Gaze of Retrospect"

Both Rieff's memoir and Leibovitz's photographs unmask Sontag's struggle with cancer in ways that the subject might find objectionable were she alive. But can their intimate, vivid depictions be construed as unethical? Does Rieff invite readers to judge his mother harshly for her death denial, or is he simply amazed at its perseverance? Is he *too* graphic in his representation of her suffering? Or do his revelations that his mother called out to him in her final hours and invested in him sole authority to choose her burial site implicitly bestow her blessing upon his literary representation of her cancer experience? Likewise, might Leibovitz's painful photographs of Sontag's illness and death entice viewers across a line between empathy and voyeurism? Does she produce "carnival images" that objectify Sontag, as Rieff alleges, or exploit Sontag in an attempt to establish herself as artist rather than commercial photographer, as some reviewers contend? (150).[12] Or do the years of intimacy the women shared and Leibovitz's revelation that she and Sontag collaborated on earlier cancer photographs imply the subject's consent to have later traumatic images taken, published, and exhibited? If reader-viewers grant that consent is not an issue, because it can be assumed or is either unknowable or irrelevant, what about audience complicity: how "should" we respond to Rieff's account of Sontag's death throes, to Leibovitz's images of her swollen corpse, especially given Sontag's caveat that "no 'we' should be taken for granted when the subject is looking at other people's pain"? (*Regarding the Pain of Others*, 7).

One ethical task of writer, photographer, and reader-viewers of cancer narratives is to act as witnesses whose empathic engagement serves, in Hirsch's words, to "enlarge the postmemorial circle" (251).[13] I am inclined to view both Leibovitz's photographs and Rieff's memoir as commemorating Sontag in an ethical manner because their representations bear unflinching, loving witness to her struggle with cancer—and because their representations move readers and viewers; help us mourn Sontag, our own beloved dead, our mortal selves; and make us stronger for having confronted the specter of loss. As Sontag notes in *Regarding the Pain of Others,* however, it is not necessarily desirable to be moved if we respond sentimentally or self-servingly to "proclaim our own innocence as well as our impotence" in the face of horror; the question is what we *do* with the knowledge traumatic photographs bring, an issue of spectatorial accountability that Rosemarie Garland-Thomson raises in *Staring* by proposing an ethics of looking: "If starers can identify with starees [*sic*] enough to jumpstart a sympathetic response that is then 'translated into action,' staring turns the corner toward the ethical" (Sontag, *Regarding the Pain of Others,* 102; Garland-Thomson, *Staring,* 185–86). Politically engaged beholding of images of women dying from cancer bears particular significance in contemporary U.S. culture, given the prevalence of the breast cancer marketplace with its infantilizing gifts of teddy bears and toys and its "ultrafeminine themes" (to use Barbara Ehrenreich's phrase)—all emphasizing sentimentality over radical activism (44). "Let me die of anything but suffocation by the pink sticky sentiment embodied in that teddy bear," Ehrenreich begs the gods and her rampaging cells (45). While there are ten million cancer survivors in the United States today whom we all can celebrate, more than two hundred forty thousand women are diagnosed annually with breast cancer, and forty thousand per year die of it; many thousands more die annually of lung, ovarian, and uterine cancers, as well as blood cancers caused by chemotherapies necessitated by earlier cancers, as Sontag did.[14] Those dying of breast cancer deserve our visual and political activism; those dead from cancer deserve not to be forgotten. Leibovitz's photographs and Rieff's memoir can thus be construed as ethical because they invite viewers and readers to behold Sontag and to remember her as both a healthy, vibrant woman and an ill and dying one, for as she argued in *Regarding the Pain of Others,* "remembering *is* an ethical act, has ethical value in and of itself. Memory is, achingly, the only relation we can have with the dead. So the belief that remembering is an ethical act is deep in our natures as humans, who know we are going to die, and who mourn those who in the normal course of things die before us" (115).[15] While she goes on to note that "too much remembering (of ancient grievances: Serbs, Irish) embitters," Sontag urges that commemorating the dead be accompanied by penetrating cultural reflection on why and how visual

and verbal depictions of them matter, for while there is no such thing as
collective memory, "there is collective instruction," and "there's nothing
wrong with standing back and thinking" (85, 115, 118).

Readers and viewers might further evaluate the ethics of Rieff's memoir and Leibovitz's photographs through the lens of Sontag's commentary regarding the effects that encountering images of the Holocaust had
upon her as a child and subsequently as a philosopher. In *On Photography* Sontag analyzes her experience of a "negative epiphany" at age twelve
when she found in a bookstore photographic images of concentration
camp survivors.

> What good was served by seeing them? They were only photo-
> graphs—of an event I had scarcely heard of and could do nothing
> to affect, of suffering I could hardly imagine and could do nothing
> to relieve. When I looked at those photographs, something broke.
> Some limit had been reached, and not only that of horror; I felt
> irrevocably grieved, wounded but a part of my feelings started to
> tighten; something went dead; something is still crying. (20)

The process described here—breakage, wounds, limit-setting, numbness, and perpetual howling—depicts the conflict that Sontag considers
inevitable for viewers of traumatic images, which compel even as they
risk anesthetizing. In the words of Griselda Pollock, the young Sontag
responded in a manner "typical as a defence against the threat of the
traumatic image," as "a certain withdrawal or an overaffectivity floods
the viewing subject" ("Dying, Seeing, Feeling," 224). Yet these numbing
images moved her over many years: "something is still crying" (Sontag,
On Photography, 20).

Pollock's theory explains further the haunting power and ethical contexts of images of trauma. The ethical involves our relation to an other,
and images of humans at their moment of most extreme vulnerability
demand that viewers consider not only what such images might do *to*
us but also what they might "do *for* both us and the other across time
and space," as part of the work of cultural mourning and remembering
(Pollock, "Dying, Seeing, Feeling," 235). To explore these issues Pollock
employs the discourse of Israeli artist Bracha L. Ettinger, whose parents
were Holocaust survivors and whose commemorative montage paintings
invite viewers to "encounter the ethical as the gaze of retrospect" (Pollock, "Dying, Seeing, Feeling," 214).[16] This "matrixial gaze," as Ettinger

terms it, resembles neither the appropriative, fetishizing male gaze that Laura Mulvey critiques in her classic essay "Visual Pleasure and Narrative Cinema" nor the Orphic gaze of mastery that Ettinger refutes in her acclaimed Eurydice paintings (Ettinger, 116–17; Mulvey, 6). Rather, Ettinger's work encourages "a different kind of scopic encounter with the trauma of the other," a space of intersubjectivity that foregrounds the viewer's responsibility to the image and the other-in-trauma (Pollock, "Dying, Seeing, Feeling," 227). Through a profound act of reciprocal witness—what Pollock terms "an ethical move of co- and trans-subjectivity"—spectatorship can be transformed: "The sharing of the humanity of others or the dehumanizing pain of others can be invoked in us by the creation of a threshold, a border-space that never collapses, never closes" (232–35). Although Rieff's and Leibovitz's disturbing images of Sontag's death from cancer are not comparable to representations of genocide, they do depict the trauma of an other and thus invite an ethical form of homage, a memorializing gesture that Ettinger terms "wit(h)nessing," a space of affiliation that affirms the "impossibility of not sharing" (147–48).[17]

Leibovitz's photographic sequences and Rieff's memoir perform significant cultural work that fosters interconnection. These narratives challenge the victim-blaming ideologies that Sontag critiqued in *Illness as Metaphor* and instead offer empowering representations of an ill woman's exceptional life and a dying woman's struggle, grounded in the authority of lived experience. In addition, Leibovitz's and Rieff's narratives facilitate individual, familial, and cultural mourning for one woman who died of cancer—Susan Sontag—and by extension for the hundreds of thousands of others who succumbed similarly, for intersubjective cancer narratives commemorate the ill, the dying, and the dead even as they help the living cope. Such narratives also invite reader-viewers to engage in what S. Lochlann Jain has termed an "elegiac politics": a communal, activist response to the corporate-driven, exploitative elements of breast cancer culture, a "retrieval of affect and death and illness in the context of profit" ("Cancer Butch," 506).[18] Moreover, Leibovitz's photographs of Sontag and Rieff's memoir present graphically the anger, fear, and grief with which a dying subject and her loved ones must contend, thus posing a needed corrective to death denial or to facile idealizations of the cancer experience. These narratives should therefore be subject to comparable ethical scrutiny: I see no legitimate reason for Rieff's autobiographical depiction of Sontag's death to be widely praised by reviewers as "intelligent," "movingly written . . . elegant and pained," "power[ful] beyond mere eulogy, elegy, or complaint" while Leibovitz's photographic depiction is widely castigated as "an unconscious exercise in ego gratification," "shocking in [its] intimacy," "morally vulnerable," and devoid of "considerations of taste and decency."[19] Instead, readers and viewers who travel alongside either Leibovitz or Rieff should be viewed as privileged to experience intersubjective encounters with another suffering human "in which trauma is carried, processed, and remembered" (Pollock, "Dying, Seeing, Feeling," 234). From my scholarly perspective both narratives provide tender, eloquent, and ethical commemoration; they evoke a transformational mode of spectatorship characterized not by voyeurism but by compassionate witness.

7 | Bodies, Witness, Mourning
Reading Breast Cancer Autothanatography

The critical term *autothanatography* is in one sense redundant, for as Susanna Egan acknowledges in *Mirror Talk: Genres of Crisis in Contemporary Autobiography,* "the spectre of death hovers over all autobiography, usually unnamed" (196). However, in breast cancer memoirs written by women whose disease has metastasized to stage four and whose demise seems imminent, death's spectral presence emerges as central to the narrative in ways potentially problematic for both writer and reader. As Egan notes, autothanatographers wrestle with existential as well as textual questions.

> How does one represent the unrepresentable? And why? . . . How does one connect representation of living persons to representation of their dying bodies so as to persuade a reading public that this profoundly disturbing experience is not obscene? How to make narrative sense of a body that is intrusive because often in pain and a time whose anticipated trajectory has been radically foreshortened? (195–97)

Unrepresentable moments of psychological crisis or bodily abjection, potentially intrusive textual renderings of suffering, subsequent loss or gain of textual control, and ethical conflicts of open self-disclosure versus "obscene" confession pervade life writing about deathward dissolution. In this form of autobiography the narrator often wavers between subject-in-process and subject-in-erasure, an anxiety-producing position. Moreover, as Egan observes, any reading public that engages autothanatography "has its own fear to contend with and its tendency to avoidance or denial, self-protective forms of resistance that say 'not me,' 'not really,' 'not yet'" (197). Hence readers may resist autothanatography or respond with voyeurism or horror, despite the dying memoirist's desire to avoid conjuring it.

Nonetheless, when narrators and audiences engage life writing about dying in ways that are mutually respectful, perhaps even mutually constitutive, they collaborate, implicitly or explicitly, in the production of textual and testimonial agency. The results of such collaborations are narratives of suffering and witness that Arthur Kleinman describes as *transactional,* Arthur Frank as *interhuman,* and Egan as *dialogic* (cited in Egan, 197). In *Mirror Talk* Egan summarizes well the distinctive features of autothanatography: "Dialogic forms of narrative juxtapose the disappearing act of lived experience and the production of the record so that the autothanatographer is restored from fading body into the community of text even at that most singular moment, 'in the face of death'" (198). Through polyvocality, reciprocal mirroring, readerly identification, and textual restoration, a reader-writer contract can evolve via narrative "co-respondence" (3). Einat Avrahami makes a similar point in *The Invading Body* by arguing that as readers witness "the materiality of bodily transformation and deterioration," they confront their own "moral and rhetorical complicity" with text and writer (133). Furthermore, since time elapses between moments of writing and moments of reading, readers of autothanatography are frequently aware that the writer has died although the subject-in-representation lives on. Hence reader and narrator together engage a textually embodied presence even as the reader recognizes the subject's corporeal absence. Granting a dead or dying subject discursive legitimacy and existential meaning thus requires textual collaboration.[1]

Two British journalists who published feature articles and subsequent memoirs about living with and dying of breast cancer, Ruth Picardie and Dina Rabinovitch, illustrate well the restoration from fading embodiment to communal textuality. Their writing forms the basis for this chapter, which probes the interweaving of medical, maternal, and sartorial discourses as these writers chronicle for an avid reading public their final months of life.[2] Picardie's seven columns for *Observer Life* magazine, published in the weeks before her death in September 1997, recount her struggle to reframe breast cancer as but one of her embodied identities. In these essays she employs a narrative voice understandably anguished on the one hand, surprisingly hilarious on the other, as she explores the intersections of corporeality, motherhood, and terminal illness. Picardie's memoir, *Before I Say Goodbye: Reflections and Observations from One Woman's Final Year,* is a hybrid text composed of her magazine columns, emails to and from family and friends, letters from readers, and posthumous tributes by her husband and sister, the book's editors. This collaborative narrative documents the memoirist's ravaged body, resilient psyche, and eventual death via narrative strategies of strategic self-exposure, polyvocal textuality, and communal memorialization.

Rabinovitch's 2004–7 columns in the *Guardian,* along with the memoir published shortly before her death in October 2007—*Take Off Your Party Dress: When Life's Too Busy for Breast Cancer*—and her fundraising blog, "Take Off Your Running Shoes," illuminate the shifting autobiographical, cultural, and memorializing contours that have shaped postmillennial breast cancer narratives. Unlike Picardie, Rabinovitch challenges medical hegemonies and pink-washing in ways that reflect shifts within the feminist breast cancer movement from awareness to resistance. In addition, by representing her experience of metastatic breast cancer as publicly as well as privately meaningful, Rabinovitch employs what S. Lochlann Jain terms an "elegiac politics," an analytical framework that "argues for pushing the private face of cancer cultures—grief, anger, death, and loss into the public cultures of cancer" ("Living in Prognosis," 89).

Shifting Corporeal Identities: Ruth Picardie's Last Will
and Testament

What is at stake for writer and readers in confronting autobiographical representations of dying bodies? In *Lost Bodies: Exploring the Borders of Life and Death* Laura E. Tanner argues that "thinking about the body in the context of mortality" reveals its liminal status and complicates the cultural contexts in which it circulates. "Although we cannot talk about the body outside the mediating discourses within which it is culturally constructed," Tanner explains, "we cannot, at the same time, disentangle knowledge or perception from the living-moving body through which we experience the world" (7). If ill bodies have long been "lost to cultural view," as she contends, then memoirs of terminal illness reinstate somatic visibility and invite readers to affirm a living body even as a narrator describes its disintegration (2).

Picardie's representation of the multiple, contingent bodies that she inhabits as a metastatic breast cancer patient can be analyzed through a series of questions that Sidonie Smith poses in a valuable essay on women autobiographers and embodiment, "Identity's Body." The first questions—"Whose body is speaking?" and "What are the implications for subjectivity of the body's positioning?"—can be used to illuminate Picardie's narrative representations of medicalization following her diagnosis and subsequent unsuccessful treatments, including chemotherapy, radiation, and various holistic therapies (271). Picardie's first *Observer Life* column of June 22, 1997, juxtaposes an account of her stable relational and professional life before breast cancer with the unstable future she confronts upon learning that her disease has metastasized. The narrator's use of direct address via the second-person pronoun *you,* followed immediately by a shift to the first-person plural *we,* invites reader identification.

> You're 32, a stone-and-a-half overweight . . . but, still, life is pretty great: you've got a husband who can make squid ink pasta and has all his own hair, your one-year-old twins are sleeping through the night and, as for your career—well, you might be interviewing George Clooney next week.
>
> And that lump in your left breast, the one you noticed after you stopped breastfeeding last summer? . . . your lump, I'm sorry to say, is actually cancer. Or should we say lumps, because, oops, it's spread to the lymph nodes under your arm and in your neck, which means it's stage three cancer and you've a 50:50 chance of living five years. (44)

Picardie portrays vividly how a metastatic breast cancer diagnosis disrupts domestic contentment, forecloses professional opportunities, and erases any presumption of a normal life span. As if these concerns were not troubling enough, the narrator further acknowledges having recently learned of her liver and lung metastases: "Abruptly, you enter the bleakly euphemistic world of palliative care. Pollyanna commits suicide" (45). This stark rendition of quick movement from diagnosis to palliation stuns readers, and shock might well turn to voyeurism were it not for Picardie's implicit invitation to respond as reciprocal witnesses to the unfolding crisis of a medicalized subject-in-process.

Any hope readers amass that alternative therapies or massive chemotherapy might improve Picardie's prognosis dissolves upon encountering the opening paragraph of her August 3, 1997, *Observer Life* column, in which she reveals further metastasis.

> It's official, then. After nine months of talking bravely about 50:50 survival rates . . . of bone disease being a really "good" form of secondary breast cancer . . . of a new, "natural" chemotherapy regime which is showing really promising results . . . of confident declarations of recovery from my healer and Chinese doctor . . . I now have a brain tumour. . . . So no more false dawns, no more miracle cures, no more *Alien*-style eruptions of disease (I now have a "full house" of secondary breast cancer sites—or "mets," as we professionals like to say). The bottom line is, I'm dying. (68)

In this passage Picardie unmasks the optimistic discourses of both Western and Eastern medical practitioners who have purveyed false hope despite her cancer's spread. While her chatty tone, wry appropriation of medical colloquialisms, and casual presentation of a devastating prognosis initially deflect attention from the seriousness of her plight, Picardie's final proclamation—"I'm dying"—positions her narrative subjectivity as that of a terminal cancer patient.

As Picardie disavows once more her internal Pollyanna, she wrenches the fantasy of miraculous recovery away from readers as well. While she claims not to be surprised by her brain tumor, since she has experienced frequent severe headaches, she admits fearing that she is "going bonkers" despite her oncologist's explanation that her brain's affected right frontal lobe is not essential to cognition (69). His subsequent reassurance that "the liver disease is going to get [you] before the brain tumour" comforts her in a macabre way (69). After outlining for readers the effects of secondary liver cancer—nausea, appetite and weight loss, extreme itching, jaundice, and severe pain—Picardie finds only slight solace: "Turning into a bruised lemon is, I reckon, better than going mad" (69). As a critically ill speaking subject with tumors in every major organ, she represents her breast cancer body as incurable and delivers that news to readers in an elegiac yet witty manner.

An additional question that Smith raises in "Identity's Body" is relevant to Picardie's textual presentation of her disrupted maternal body: "What are the strategic purposes and uses around which the body has been autobiographically mobilized?" (272). A grieving maternal discourse devoid of self-pity is evident in her first *Observer Life* column, in which she confides her bone metastasis and diagnostic shift to stage-four breast cancer. At that point, Picardie explains, both she and her physician begin to rationalize.

> Your oncologist tells you that this is the "best" secondary breast cancer to have, because the skeleton isn't a vital organ and you can live with it for years. . . . As for not seeing your babies grow up, better to have had half a life with your beautiful children than a whole life without. (45)

Readers immediately recognize, however, that secondary cancers are life-threatening and that as the mother of infant twins, the writer has enjoyed not half a lifetime with her babies but merely a year. Picardie turns to gallows humor in her third column, published a month later, complaining that "having a terminal illness is supposed to make you extremely wise and evolved, turning you into the kind of person who thinks, 'What is being 11 stone compared with the joy of seeing my children run through a flowery meadow as if in a junior Timotei ad?' Unfortunately, I just can't get my head around Zen meditation" (57–58). This wry representation of children as imaginary advertisement fodder wards off reader pity, even as the writer challenges culturally sanctioned visions of a terminally ill woman's capacity for maternal transcendence.[3]

Picardie's deflection of sympathy through humor dissipates in her next *Observer Life* essay, in which she confronts the secondary cancer that has invaded her brain. In this August 3, 1997, column the writer mobilizes her maternal body as a site of mourning.

> What hurts most is losing the future. I won't be there to clap when my beloved babies learn to write their names; I won't see them learn to swim, or go to school, or play the piano; I won't be able to read them *Pippi Longstocking,* or kiss their innocent knees when they fall off their bikes. (69)

This litany of lost maternity evokes death's power to snatch the writer's future, as she laments her coming absence from her children's daily lives. To be sure, Picardie briefly turns again to mordant humor in an attempt to undercut her anguish: "(All right, so I won't have to clean pooh out of the bath, or watch *Pingu* for the 207th time, or hose spinach sauce off the floor.") (69). However, as she writes about preparing memory boxes for her twins, Lola and Joe, Picardie evokes her readers' emotional identification and invites compassionate witness: "How do you write the definitive love letter to a partly imaginary child?" (69–70).

This question haunts Picardie's friends and readers, as is evident in their letters reassuring her that the children will remember her. A friend identified as Carrie insists to Picardie via email,

> I have done some reflecting on the issue of J&L's memories of you. I am not saying this to make you feel better. But I think they will remember you. Firstly, I remember before I was 2—I have memories that nobody would ever have bothered suggesting to me because of their complete banality. . . . Secondly, you are so central to their little lives that they will ask about you constantly, and be shown photos and videos and you will be talked about. (63)

Observer Life reader Sarah Briggs assures Picardie that her children will come to know her through her columns: "*I have just read your article in the Observer and felt I must write to you—don't worry if you are unable to compile memory boxes for your beautiful children—just make sure someone keeps this article for them and they will understand and know what a wonderful person their mother is*" (71). And reader Susanna Harris affirms, "*Your kids will always know what a special mother they had. Scant consolation, I know, for not being there. But life is cruel at times, and there's no point in avoiding that fact. Your memory will stay alive forever, in your Matthew's mind, in that of your friends . . . And the tales that everyone tells will build up a picture for your kids. And that will help them*" (74). Picardie's forthright discussion of anticipated maternal loss thus facilitates communal witness.

Another question from Smith's essay "Identity's Body," "Is the autobiographical body being given to the reader, or withheld?", can be usefully applied to Picardie's narrative use of sartorial discourses, as she confesses an obsession with negative body image exacerbated by her breast cancer diagnosis and treatment (272). A comical discussion of finding appropriate clothes after gaining weight from medications begins early in Picardie's *Observer Life* columns, alongside an evolving addiction to therapeutic shopping. In her July 27, 1997, column she complains that while "everybody thinks cancer makes you thin . . . I'm getting fatter and fatter" and describes her daily garb as "clever Ghost clothes with elasticated waists"; in a subsequent column she admits that "it's bloody tough living in limbo, not knowing exactly how long I've got left," then deflects her worry by asking rhetorically, "Can I justify going to the next Ghost sale, and who gets my black skirt after my death?" (57, 70). In these passages Picardie employs mordant humor and seduces readers who can identify with her gendered bodily angst.

Picardie offers further sartorial confession in a column published four weeks before her death, in which she jokingly extols consumerism as an antidote to despair: "After months of careful research, I have discovered a treatment that is a) cheaper than complementary therapy; b) a hell of a lot more fun than chemotherapy, and c) most important, incredibly effective! Retail therapy!" (90). Despite a bounced credit card and a swollen brain, the writer feigns relief that her "other problem—my enlarged liver—I believe has been solved by my later splurge at Whistles sale (blue skirt, lilac shirt). Even if the dread organ doesn't shrink, the clever bias cutting hides most of the lumps" (91). At the end of this column she asks her audience to stay tuned for publication of a self-help book she is writing, *Shop Yourself Out of Cancer*. As these examples attest, Picardie uses strategic exaggeration to shift readers' attention from metastases to fashion dilemmas.

This self-deprecating discourse of clothing consumption occurs as well in email exchanges with friends that are incorporated into *Before I Say Goodbye*. In a February 25, 1997, email to India, for instance, Picardie confides plans for an upcoming holiday with her husband—"FIRST NIGHT WITHOUT THE KIDS"—and admits that she "blew 425 pounds on underwear (including stomach hiding silk slip) from Agent Provocateur" (24). Although she acknowledges this purchase as excessive, she justifies it as a distraction from her prognosis and an affirmation of her marriage: "Stupid, or what? But I look like such a slob most of the time, and Matt will be so excited and, what the fuck, I'm dying. You can wear it after I've kopped it. Bye!" Picardie signs off "From a Pig," signaling both her worry about weight gain and her pleasure in having exceeded the boundaries of retail propriety. In subsequent emails to India, Picardie describes herself as "busy finding my inner Shallow Fashion Bimbo before I die," reassures her friend that "you ALWAYS look fabulously well-groomed, chic, elegant, stylish and make me feel even more like an overgrown student," and again extols the distraction of shopping.

My life as a fashion bimbo continues: yesterday bought pair of linen trousers (elasticized waist) and linen shirt from Hobbs (my new favourite shop, though size 16 jacket was too tight) and new pair of (brown, three strap) Birkenstocks. What is happening to me? But it is such good therapy. I wish summer would hurry up: I never know what shoes to wear in the winter. (29–31)

The irony of a dying woman wishing time would speed up rather than stand still, merely for the sake of easier shoe selection, evokes readers' elegiac laughter, as does the speaker's wry sartorial detail.

The fact that Picardie did not live to see her columns, letters, and emails published in *Before I Say Goodbye* raises issues discussed here regarding the ethics of representation (chapters 5 and 6, this volume). The posthumous publication of private emails—a decision made by Picardie's husband and sister but with the agreement of the authors—invites the question of whether Picardie's permission was ever sought and granted. In his foreword Seaton assures readers that Picardie wanted her emails and letters included should her memoir ever be published: "Ruth knew she had left a rich resource of writing in her e-mail correspondence—in fact, it was her idea that any book of hers might include a selection from them. In compiling this book, I know that we have been carrying out her wishes" (ix). Readers can thus conclude that Picardie endorsed *Before I Say Goodbye* as a project of self-memorialization.[4] A further aspect of the book's memorializing capacities is the inclusion of a final *Observer Life* column by Justine Picardie that announces her sister's death and an afterword by Seaton that shares details of his wife's last days. Readers learn from Justine Picardie that Ruth entered hospice, "confined to a wheelchair, and very weak" but still engaging with her family and noticing "the small things that make people happy yet are too often forgotten: the colour of a bright lipstick, the scent of late-flowering sweet peas, the pleasure of a newly-planted pot of lavender" (106–7). Justine further testifies to Ruth's ultimate inability "to breathe without oxygen, choked by the obscene tumours that had invaded every part of her brave body," and to her sister's peaceful face immediately after dying, "though her eyebrows were raised in a slightly quizzical manner: as if to say, how can this be?" (107). Seaton's commentary reveals his wife's sporadic bouts with dementia, her alternating modes of gentleness and willfulness, and his own suffering as Picardie distanced herself from him, often angrily labeling him her "gaoler," as a wrenching but "a necessary part of letting go" (128–29). As witnesses to Seaton's grim testimony, readers wrestle with both the ethics of his revelation and the validity of his claim "that the true meaning of dying is its absolute loneliness"—an assertion mitigated by his subsequent acknowledgment that Picardie's children remain "her piece of the future," by the communal nature of Picardie's columns and emails, and by the dialogic autothanatography that is ultimately published (129–31).

As Kelly Oliver has argued, witnessing is "the constitutive event and process" of human subjectivity (17). Reader identification with Picardie's narrated life and death thus evokes an ethical encounter with the subjectivity of another human facing the abyss, as we must all eventually do. Such encounters induce a collaborative form of witness that in Oliver's view "is the heart of the circulation of energy that connects us, and obligates us, to each other" (20). Although such interconnections circulate powerfully in Picardie's memoir, they remain more personal than political. Her testimony does not critique hegemonic medical practices, question the economics of the breast cancer marketplace, or challenge mainstream cancer culture.[5] As we shall see, comparing Picardie's memoir to Rabinovitch's highlights differences in cultural perspective between premillennial and postmillennial autothanatographies.

Shifting Cultural Contours: Dina Rabinovitch's
Dying Words

A London-based journalist who specialized in children's literature and family issues, a wife-mother-stepmother at the center of a blended family with eight children ranging in age from two to nineteen, and an Ashkenazi Jew with strongly held Orthodox beliefs and close ties to Israel, Rabinovitch was diagnosed in 2004 at forty-one with an aggressive form of estrogen-negative, stage-three breast cancer. From September 2004 through August 2005 she wrote a fortnightly features column for the *Guardian*, "Getting to Know the Enemy Within," that candidly chronicled her cancer experience, attracted thousands of readers, and received journalistic acclaim. As her health declined over the next two years Rabinovitch provided update articles for the *Guardian;* published the memoir *Take Off Your Party Dress*, a revised, expanded version of her columns; and began a fund-raising blog that she entitled "Take Off Your Running Shoes." The final posting on her blog, a personal and cultural lamentation entitled "We've Seen Wars, We've Seen Plagues, but Never This," appeared a week before she died in October 2007; it began, "There is no template for the way I am living now" (www.guardian.co.uk).

An additional theoretical question that Sidonie Smith explores in "Identity's Body" can help readers probe the contingent modes of bodily identity that Rabinovitch represents: "What specific body does the autobiographical subject claim in her text?" (271). As with Picardie's narratives, Rabinovitch's columns and memoir present maternal, sartorial, and medicalized bodies in discursive registers that range from witty to grief-stricken. Rabinovitch's narrative differs from Picardie's, however, in its use of outrage—at the British medical establishment's experimental treatments on stage-four patients despite virtually no hope of remission, at breast cancer culture's crass displays of October pink, at widespread cultural silence about the reality that mothers everywhere are dying even as their daughters, sisters, and friends don ribbons and run races.

As an autobiographical subject Rabinovitch claims a maternal body that is familial as well as culturally inscribed. As the nursing mother of a son, Elon, who is almost three when she is diagnosed with breast cancer yet who still enjoys a nightly dose of "meee," his word for breast milk, and a mother-stepmother to other young children who wander into the room when she is bathing or disrobing, Rabinovitch recognizes her precancer body as not entirely her own. Her narrative recounts moments prior to her diagnosis in which she has happily given her breast to Elon for nourishment and has comfortably exposed her body to domestic observation. Breast cancer represents a major rupture in these mutually pleasurable acts of corporeal revelation. The surgeon who diagnoses her, having probed in alarm her 7-centimeter "Tony Soprano of lumps," insists that she stop breast-feeding immediately and sends her home after biopsy with her breast bandaged yet oozing, too painful to be touched (25). A huge part of Rabinovitch's embodied maternal identity must therefore shift, given her earlier claim that "I can breast-feed anywhere, and have done, including on top of a camel in the Sinai desert" and her prior delight in conversing unclothed with her children during their bathroom forays (15).

Rabinovitch's early representation of her maternal body as a source of agency and nurture is complicated by her uneasy admission that she did not heed her body's warnings. She acknowledges to her consulting breast surgeon, and subsequently to readers, that although she found a small lump during pregnancy, she did not consult a doctor until three years later, when it "felt like a rectangular slab of metal embedded inside" (7). When she asks her surgeon, "I should have come earlier, shouldn't I, childlike, seeking dispensation," both she and we as readers are relieved that he "offers it instantly. 'We don't talk about what's already happened, no, no, no, it's closed'" (2). What distracted Rabinovitch from investigating the lump were the bodily rhythms of pregnancy and lactation and a complex domestic life with an infant and seven other children, not to mention marriage and a multifaceted journalistic career. Post-diagnosis, Rabinovitch's embodied identity and her household routines change of necessity. She describes, for example, her anguish at telling Elon that she can't feed him anymore when he cries "I only want meee," and she recounts her dismay at finding her ten-year-old daughter weeping in the bathroom after her mother loses her hair from chemotherapy, afraid that her hair too is thinning (71, 86).

In narrating her struggles with sartorial as well as maternal embodiment, Rabinovitch scrutinizes her breast cancer body's subjection to public and private gazes. She often does this humorously through a pragmatic focus on fashion issues for the post-mastectomy woman, from how to choose a party dress that deemphasizes her one-breasted status to which types of organic cotton are comfortable enough not to irritate her irradiated chest. A recurring issue is what an ill woman wears when being photographed, as she often was while conducting interviews with Philip Pullman or Madonna and attending public functions as the wife of a prominent London attorney: "I am now adamant that I don't want clothes that fake it. I want a look that works with the reality of my body. Not the 'cumfie'—soft, foam-filled stuffing for the gap in my bra" (129). Rabinovitch also recounts amusing sartorial anecdotes about her children: a teenaged daughter's text message that reveals discomfort with her mother's baldness ("Pls, Mum, can U wear hat to pick me up. XXX"); her toddler son's glee at pulling down the neckline of his mother's carefully selected bathing suit to reveal her breastless chest to an astounded lifeguard. Although she admits occasionally desiring to conceal her one-breastedness, Rabinovitch's narrative self-disclosure publicly affirms her breast cancer body.

Another question that Smith raises in "Identity's Body"—"Where is the body narratively to be found and how does it circulate through the text?"—resonates in Rabinovitch's memoir as well (271). A survey of the narrative body's representation in Take Off Your Party Dress reveals a catalog of adjectives whose connotative weight threatens to strip agency

from the speaking subject: *flat, scarred, skewed, foggy, battered*. Yet Rabinovitch also proffers a post-mastectomy counterdiscourse composed of
present participles that connote embodied vitality: *healing, writing, cook-
ing, shopping, interviewing*. Through use of a strategically fluid autobiographical lexicon she affirms multiple, if contingent, embodied identities.

Two additional questions from Smith's essay—"How is the body the
performative boundary between . . . the subject and the world?" and
"What kind of performance is the body allowed to give?"—provide a
useful framework for analyzing Rabinovitch's narrative representation of
medicalization (272). She begins her memoir by recounting the circumstances of her diagnosis and personalizing her surgeon, Mr. Al-Dubaisi,
whose assistance in translating unfamiliar medical discourse she appreciates and whom she playfully compares to the Old Testament patriarch
Abraham; she appreciates his sensitivity to bodily privacy in covering
her left breast when he examines her right and his sigh upon realizing
that his nurse neglected to do this already. Bodily concealment and revelation feature prominently throughout the narrative, as Rabinovitch
interrogates breast cancer's public spaces and recounts her experience
of mastectomy, radiation, chemotherapy, multiple recurrences, experimental drug trials, and skin and bone metastases. In both columns and
memoir she argues that private/public boundaries shrink when a breast
cancer patient is infantilized, her body a site of surveillance. In the 2005
column "One Year On," for example, she echoes Ehrenreich in discussing
how medical practitioners and even family members strip her of agency:
"It is, above all, infantilizing to have a life-threatening illness," to find
one's identity transformed from being an all-singing, all-dancing mom,
"to being labeled with this mortal sickness that makes everybody lower
their voice before they get to the end of the word can-cer, so the second syllable comes out in a reverent hush" (171). To resist objectification
Rabinovitch mobilizes her body as a force to contend with. In a memoir
chapter on metastasis, for example, she describes an angry chest covered
in swollen lesions: "I can see the cancer growing. It's on my chest wall, I
can see the red patches" (241). This line depicts an alien but potent body
in which cancer has literally surfaced—a traumatized site that garners
physicians' amazement and defies infantilization by "speaking" harsh somatic truth.[6]

Although Rabinovitch rarely expresses direct anger at her oncologists
or at the research scientists whom she consults while participating in
drug trials, she acknowledges that often "all I get is an incredibly battered

feeling, and I leave in tears" and recounts confronting one specialist with her vulnerable body's full force: "I feel like I'm in a dark room . . . and you're all chucking apples at me, hoping one will hit home" (253–54). In passages such as these she questions medical hegemony despite acknowledging the limitations of available treatments for metastatic cancers. In addition, she indicts pharmaceutical companies for marketing lucrative targeted breast cancer treatments rather than sponsoring cause-seeking research, and she notes that one renowned physician acknowledged her critique: "'It's commercial,' Dr de Bono says. 'The drugs companies won't put money into diagnosing the structures of tumours, only into cures'" (254). The physician's calm then shifts to outrage: "You can make a profit, you see, out of 'curing' people; they pay for the medicine. Work out the cause, though, and they may not need the medicine after all" (254). Confronted with economic injustice, the frustrated narrator describes sobbing uncontrollably as she leaves the hospital: "I shouldn't have come on my own" (254).[7]

Despite moments of despair, Rabinovitch is never passive in the face of medicalization; she questions the efficacy of many procedures even when submitting to them. Having agreed to genetic testing, for example, because her maternal grandmother and several cousins died of breast cancer, she expressed skepticism about her negative test results—"I don't trust the genetic screen"—although she is relieved that the alleged outcome is "good news for my daughters" (199). Having endured the side effects of several drug trials, she accuses her oncologist of experimenting on a generation of women much as physicians did during the thalidomide era fifty years before and responds ambivalently to his reply that enrollment in trials does not constitute experimentation as long as a patient might be helped. At times Rabinovitch disarms readers with humor at her physicians' expense, as when she admits that to distract herself from her dying body she "wonders how these doctors are when they confront their partners' breasts in bed," a fantasy that represents physicians as vulnerable and enhances her narrative agency (221). At the same time she confesses her own embodied vulnerability: "I find myself obsessively checking the Nottingham Prognostic Index, a calculating tool you can read on the Internet, by which you multiply the grade of your tumour by 0.2 and add the stage of your cancer . . . and then you can find out whether your chemotherapy is going to work or not. Or something" (226). Near the end of her memoir she recounts dismay at having entered "the outer edges of cancer treatment," a phrase her physicians use too often (258). In such passages Rabinovitch chronicles the anxiety that accompanies the threshold space of mortal unknowing that Jain has termed "living in prognosis" (Jain, "Living in Prognosis," 77–78).

Another strategic purpose for which Rabinovitch's narrative mobilizes her dying body is to assess the value of an individual life. This terminally ill woman's anguished negotiation of the boundaries between self and world is evident in a June 8, 2006, column (later incorporated into her memoir) entitled "What Is My Life Worth?" After answering this question—"seventy-five thousand and eighty-five pounds, and fourteen pence"—she wryly identifies the sum as "the cost of my treatment to date" (220). This calculation of the economics of cancer echoes the ethical scrutiny in an earlier column, "One Year On," of her class privilege as a private cancer patient: "What do you do when you know there's a life-saving drug available, but only the patients who can afford it can have it?" (www.guardian.co.uk). Acknowledging that wealth allows her private hospitals, single rooms, and expensive experimental drugs, Rabinovitch expresses guilt at her decision to seek cutting-edge treatment from famous U.S. oncologists. Dismayed that most ill women lack these privileges, she creates a blog to raise funds for patients who cannot afford care at her North London private hospital.[8]

As an autothanatographer, Rabinovitch mourns the fact that despite endless medical experiments nothing works; her remissions are brief, her tumors grow, and "increasingly, I need ever harder-core diversions to distract me from what's happening to my body" (221). To understand the narrative trajectory of her final memoir chapters and subsequent columns, we can consider Egan's questions in *Mirror Talk:* "How do people who are terminally ill think autobiographically?" (27) What narrative strategies can be used to represent a "confrontation with annihilation," the tensions of a body under erasure that nonetheless remain a "living presence"? (197–98). Rabinovitch's goals are pedagogical, testimonial, and political, as her final published column of October 22, 2007, attests. When she "check[s] out the depressingly regular obituaries," she explains, "the ages [are] always similar—46, 41, 48, leaving behind a son, a daughter, two children, maybe three"; such obituaries describe dead women's accomplishments but never explore "how, actually, one is supposed to live each day with illness" (www.guardian.co.uk). Thus Rabinovitch desanitizes her experience of dying in hopes of helping readers understand what *not* surviving breast cancer really means. To this end she catalogs ineffectual chemo cocktails prescribed by her frustrated oncologists: massive doses of Herceptin intended to combat her estrogen-negative tumor (the only effect of which is a dual recurrence); unsuccessful attempts at pharmaceutical "synergy" (a favorite medical word, she notes) through an innovative combination of Herceptin and Omnitarg; a brief flirtation with capecitabine, "a standard chemotherapy drug" that fails to shrink her tumors; and eventual enrollment in three experimental drug trials featuring first the "flaming orange" and nauseating Tykerb, then concoctions with surreal labels such as 17AAG and 17 DMeg—all injected over many months to no avail. However well she masters the spelling and side effects of "this year's magic bullet," no drug prevents her cancer's spread. Unable to master her disease or its medical discourses, Rabinovitch resorts finally to the voice of a child in tantrum: "I have it, is all I know, and I just don't want it" (www.guardian.co.uk).

In her final column Rabinovitch presents reconfigured testimonial versions of the maternal and sartorial "speaking" bodies that she conjured earlier in her memoir. These shifting representations recall an additional question from "Identity's Body," "What is the relationship of autobiographical body politics to the body politic, of individual anatomy to cultural anatomy?" (Smith, 272). In exploring the intersection between her failing body and the bodies of other dying women Rabinovitch reveals a feminist political lens, as she mourns the catastrophic death of a generation of mothers: "Mothers are being targeted by an illness, for the first time in our history, and families are losing their linchpins. We've had war, we've had plagues, but never before have we had an illness that has killed off the mothers" (www.guardian.co.uk). A mother's death undoes her family, as her description of being too ill to attend her kindergartner's awards ceremony, too nauseated to "make tuna sandwiches on days when you can't face food," and too exhausted to participate in a BBC-radio discussion of good parenting after divorce attest. In this column Rabinovitch also laments not knowing "what the boundaries of this exhaustion are, how long it will last, what I can manage within its confines" (www.guardian.co.uk). Another maternal regret, the hiring of a daily in-home child care provider, signifies her abdication of primacy in the life of her young son, yet this decision is necessary because "breast cancer, a six-year-old—even with copious older siblings—and no back-up just doesn't work" (www.guardian.co.uk). "The shifts in how we live are inexorable," Rabinovitch concludes, an assertion supported in her final column by the sad admission that Elon no longer asks at bedtime for his weary mother to read a story. In another jolting narrative moment she likens her morphine-induced hazes to the final throes of childbirth, thus comparing her dying body to her maternal one and connecting death to life's beginnings. "I spent one of the long summer nights in death's anteroom," she reports, an experience that felt strangely familiar, like "that moment toward the end of labour, but still with hours to go, when you utterly reject any lingering notion of natural childbirth and you are yelling for the epidural" (www.guardian.co.uk). As Rabinovitch dies at home family life proceeds without her, a truth that the writer (and perhaps her readers) finds paradoxically reassuring and devastating.

Despite the somber tone of this final column, Rabinovitch maintains humor to the end by offering a spirited critique of mainstream breast cancer culture. Objecting to the optimism and pink paraphernalia of Breast Cancer Awareness Month, a corporate-driven annual October event in the United Kingdom as well as the United States, she satirizes the spectacle of "pink ribbons wrapped around buildings, all manner of pink things to buy at tills—including my own bête noire, the tight-fitting T-shirts that are the antithesis of what is comfortable post-mastectomy—why, the very petrol pumps are turning pink" (www.guardian.co.uk). Still, as disturbing as she finds this sea of pink, Rabinovitch admits relief on one level that Breast Cancer Awareness Month exists. Someone needs to do *something* to stop this disease, she concludes wearily, "because too many mothers are dying" (www.guardian.co.uk).

Two final questions that Smith poses in "Identity's Body" are useful for analyzing Rabinovitch's evocation of communal witness: "Before whom is the speaker revealing/concealing . . . her body? . . . Whose history of the body is being written?" (272). Through her *Guardian* columns, memoir, and blog this journalist inscribed a public history of her breast cancer body that attracted international readers and raised more than 100,000 pounds sterling for breast cancer research. Responses by readers published after Rabinovitch's death affirm the dialogic impact of her writing. In an October 30, 2007, letter to the editor, reader Donna Anton confesses, "I burst into tears when I read that Dina Rabinovitch had died. Although she had hinted in last week's piece that the end was drawing near, I was fooled by her vigorous prose into thinking that she had more time left and we'd soon be reading about a spontaneous remission brought about by her strength of character" ("Remembering Dina," np). In a *Guardian* tribute of November 2, 2007, columnist Meg Rosoff explains that she knew Rabinovitch primarily through her writing, which sustained her as a woman whose sister had died of breast cancer and who had subsequently contracted it herself. Going public with her breast cancer felt impossible to Rosoff: "I found it far too painful and difficult even to acknowledge the process, much less document it—so I let Dina do it for me" (Rosoff, np). Whose history of the body is being written through such intersubjective exchanges? Arguably readers' histories as well as that of the writer to whom they turn for representation and inspiration.

Communal Grief and Grievability

As breast cancer mammographers, Picardie and Rabinovitch represent both their vibrant pre-diagnostic bodies—gendered, desiring, resolutely maternal—and their wounded post-diagnostic bodies. Each form of corporeality "speaks" alongside or in tandem with other bodies these writers inhabit—symbolic and temporal as well as material, public as well as private. In columns, emails, blogs, and memoirs they invite readers to witness their embodied struggles as addressees whose compassionate attention affirms the writers' narrative subjectivities—for as Oliver has argued, "witnessing as address and response is the necessary ground for subjectivity" (16). Picardie and Rabinovitch explore threshold spaces as dying women nonetheless embracing family life, as writers reflecting publicly on the internal and communal grief the prospect of their demise evokes. And as obituaries and reader letters attest, their writings have inspired a range of commemorative gestures that have generated spaces for public grieving.

Tanner's discussion in *Lost Bodies* of epistemological distinctions between grief and mourning provides a theoretical perspective for assessing autothanatography as a potential site of communal lamentation and memorialization. In exploring the U.S. cultural discomfort with ill and dying bodies, she objects to the ways mourning has traditionally been defined as a process through which to loosen the hold of the dead over the living. Reviewing dominant cultural discourses of mourning, the emotions associated with mourning in Western cultures, familiar genealogies of mourning, and mourning's ethical significance, Tanner wonders whether U.S. culture has moved "beyond mourning" (243, n. 1). Although she does not finally accept a view of mourning as culturally obsolete, she advocates "an embodied theory of loss [that] problematizes prevailing modes of mourning as emotional relinquishment. The term 'grief' seems to me less laden with cultural and theoretical assumptions that implicitly endorse existing disembodied models of loss" (243, n. 1). Breast cancer autothanatographies such as Picardie's and Rabinovitch's work against both disembodied and cultural models of mourning as emotional relinquishment by representing the fullness of dying women's embodied presence.

Judith Butler's theorization of grief, grievability, and mourning offers a final framework for assessing the potential impact of dialogic auto-thanatography. Although *Precarious Life: The Powers of Mourning and Violence* (2004) and *Frames of War: When Is Life Grievable?* (2009) focus on the cultural invisibility of victims and displaced survivors of wars and genocides, two questions Butler raises—How does a culture determine whose bodies can/should be publically grieved, and how do a culture's orthodox or resistant methods of public mourning circulate?—are relevant to any study of life writing about dying. Bodies are never really private, she contends in *Precarious Life:* "Constituted as a social phenomenon in the public sphere, my body is and is not mine. Given over from the start to the social world of others, it bears the imprint, is formed within the crucible of social life. Only later, and with some uncertainty, do I lay claim to my body as my own, if in fact I ever do" (26). A similar claim occurs in *Frames of War:* "The boundary of who I am is the boundary of the body, but the boundary of the body never fully belongs to me. Survival depends less on the established boundary to the self than on the constitutive sociability of the body" (54).

Butler further argues that public expressions of grief enact constitutive sociability: "Perhaps we can say that grief contains the possibility of apprehending a mode of dispossession that is fundamental to who I am" (*Precarious Life,* 28). Public grieving can become "a resource for politics" that enables mourners to comprehend the vulnerabilities of the dispossessed, whether violated by armed struggle or by amoral disease (30). In Butler's theorization grief "may be understood as the slow process by which we develop a point of identification with suffering itself. The disorientation of grief—'Who have I become?' or, indeed, 'What is left of me? What is it in the Other that I have lost?'—posits the 'I' in the mode of unknowingness" (37). Once mourners, and arguably once compassionate readers of autothanatography, "unknow" themselves in the face of the suffering of others, which they witness literally or vicariously, the somatic and existential "mode of unknowingness" that remains can become a public space for reciprocal witness and communal grieving. The AIDS memorial quilt (the Names Project) and HIV-AIDS vigils of the

late twentieth century served as breakthroughs in this regard, Butler suggests, by affirming that "the differential distribution of public grieving is
a political issue of enormous significance"; in contrast, the Bush administration's denial of any public grievability of the death of Iraqi citizens
at the hands of U.S. military forces provided what Butler deems an early
twenty-first-century unethical counterexample (38).[9]

Tanner and Butler remind us that public grieving, mourning, and memorializing are culturally shaped and sanctioned. As I have contended
throughout this study, one important example of the ethical stakes of that
shaping is located in the postmillennial explosion of visual and textual
breast cancer narratives, including autothanatography. What cultural
work is accomplished through such public disclosure of private suffering, and what circumstances have led women to share their breast cancer experiences, even their dying reflections, in narratives that constitute
testimonial and memorial projects? One answer lies in autothanatographers' frequent resistance to cultural myths and silences. As Martha
Nussbaum has noted, people marked by incapacitating disability or terminal illness challenge the Western "myth of the citizen as a competent
independent adult"—a fiction of invulnerability that many breast cancer
memoirists refuse to endorse; they instead create forthright narratives
that acknowledge pain and interdependency (411). Also relevant are Butler's comments on the "differential distribution of public grieving" and
the corrective model to discriminatory practices of mourning provided
by HIV/AIDS activists of the 1980s and 1990s, who claimed public exhibition space to honor the dead through images stitched together com-
munally. As of 2011 the AIDS memorial quilt contained 40,000 panels
and had attracted fourteen million viewers worldwide (www.aidsquilt.
org). Might a breast cancer memorial quilt attract equal numbers of participants and have a similar public impact?[10] Like HIV/AIDS memoirists and activists, cancer autothanatographers resist differential modes of
grieving by thrusting their dying bodies and self-memorializing projects
into a sometimes myopic public sphere—and, in some cases, by demand-
ing increased research dollars to investigate understudied causes, new
prevention strategies, promising treatments, and a viable cure for a disease
whose cultural discourses too often focus on survival without acknowledgment of those who have died. Ruth Picardie and Dina Rabinovitch are
two of many autothanatographers whose narratives evoke empathic witness and communal grieving as a means of keeping the dying subject culturally visible and gesturing toward new forms of breast cancer activism.

Afterword

What Remains

As a final consideration of the public impact of autothanatographic projects that reckon with breast cancer, let us turn to Lisa Saltzman's theories of commemorative art in *Making Memory Matter,* where she offers rich avenues for exploring "the aesthetic dimensions and the ethical capacities of visual objects that pursue the question of memory in the present" (11–12). Saltzman is interested in how and why contemporary Western cultures are "consumed by the concept, if not always the actual work of memory"; her study thus focuses on memorial art that refuses representation's fetishistic tendencies in favor of its materiality (5). Although she acknowledges the authority traditionally granted to figurative commemorative practices in sculpture and architecture, she rightly notes that Maya Lin's 1982 Vietnam Veterans Memorial has influenced cultural memory by enshrining names of dead soldiers on a black wall, "at once wound and scar," rather than portraying as representative hero an iconic soldier or martyr (8).[1] Other "postindexical" artistic strategies for marking absence and commemorating loss include animated monuments, vaudevillian silhouettes, and architectural memorials by artists such as Krzysztof Wodiczko, whose 1998 video installation *Bunker Hill Monument Project* transformed a Boston landmark into a testimonial screen enabling public viewers to mourn and remember local victims of urban violence through "prosthetic witness"; Christian Boltanski, whose 1990 public art project *Missing House* commemorated the irredeemable loss of the Eastern European Jewish immigrants who lived at 15/16 Grosse Hamburger Strasse in Berlin prior to their evacuation during the Holocaust; and Kara Walker, whose silhouettes in *Gone* (1994) parodied racist and sexually exploitative encounters during slavery and thereby forged an "ethics of spectrality" (41, 73, 93–95).[2] At its best, Saltzman contends, such work "intervenes in an amnesiac public sphere and offers up . . . the possibility of representing something of a community's history" (16). Like Susan Sontag, who claimed in *Regarding the Pain of Others* that the

"Western memory bank is mostly a visual one," Saltzman argues that because memory and visual culture are linked in postmillennial culture, it is essential to analyze the aesthetic and ethical implications of that conjunction (Sontag, 1; Saltzman, 5). Understanding cultural practices of memory such as reading aloud names of the dead or placing wreaths at sites of roadside accidents, as well as studying vigils, funerary objects, and shrines such as the Vietnam Wall, is important because they promote remembrance and call viewers to conscience.[3]

"What is the work of mourning and memory?" Saltzman wonders near the end of *Making Memory Matter*—a question essential to pose with regard to women and men worldwide who have died from breast cancer, whose deaths have too often been invisible amid the relentless optimism of U.S. cancer culture with its federally mandated Office of Survivorship and its endless pink products for sale. The photographs that I consider in this Afterword serve as insignia of remembrance and aesthetic responses to loss that have circulated through publication in anthologies or blogs and through exhibition in art galleries or museums. Charlee Brodsky's image of Stephanie Byram's abandoned running shoes in the photo-documentary *Knowing Stephanie,* Dina Rabinovitch's photograph of the fashionable gray hat she wore to temple and displayed on her "Take Off Your Running Shoes" blog shortly before her death, and Annie Leibovitz's images from *A Photographer's Life* of Susan Sontag's shell collection, abandoned manuscripts, empty apartment, and tiny silhouette poised beneath a massive funerary monument all render traces of lives lost to breast cancer that hover between indexical and iconic representation. These images serve as mute testimonials that invite viewers to engage in communal mourning and remembrance—for Byram, Rabinovitch, and Sontag and, by extension, for others whose lives have ended prematurely due to cancer.

Brodsky's decision to conclude *Knowing Stephanie* with an image of stilled running shoes enables readers to confront the loss of a vibrant subject who wished to be remembered for her joie de vivre and activism. As noted in chapter 5, Byram participated in thirty Susan G. Komen Race for the Cure runs during her last eight years and raised nearly $100,000 for breast cancer research. While the sneakers initially appear to have been posed atop a leafy landscape, their untied laces suggest that they were discarded as their owner moved off barefooted toward her next activity (which might well have required hiking boots, since Byram walked for five days through three mountain passes to visit Machu Picchu shortly before her death). Beside this final image lies a narrative reminder by Byram that while dying is inevitable, meanwhile there is living: *"What is in my future: love, laughter, gardens, family, friends, spirituality, travel . . . more of what I love in life. I surround myself with positivity, gentleness, challenge, and hope. . . . I am, until I pass, as we all shall"* (99).

As Brodsky explains in her preface, until Byram's death in 2001 the two women decided every facet of this memorial project together, including the selection of exhibition sites and the creation of a documentary film, *Stephanie: A Story of Transformation* (9).[4] In a conversation with biographer Jennifer Matesa in 2000, Byram explained the solidarity she felt with other breast cancer patients yet her resistance to cultural discourses of survival.

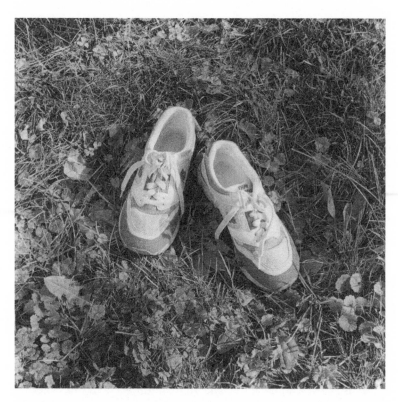

Charlee Brodsky, *Stephanie's Running Shoes*. Courtesy of the artist.

I feel a tremendous bond with other men and women who have survived the breast cancer experience. . . . It is a terrifying, lonely, sometimes shameful experience to look and feel so different, to wear the unmistakable beacons of cancer that invite total strangers to ask, "How much longer will you be in treatment?" With many women who have had cancer, . . . we exchange a glance and we suddenly skip all formalities and get to the realities: relishing today, relinquishing control, carefully budgeting our time and energy, and, most importantly, loving and laughing.

Despite this pride . . . , the word "survivor" grates on my nerves. We all live with our various misfortunes, having AIDS or osteoporosis, living without health insurance, being in bad marriages or raising difficult children. We are all survivors. Why should breast cancer be any different? (Brodsky and Byram, 124)

In this testimony Byram acknowledges sister breast cancer patients as a primary audience for her photo-narrative, yet she expands its reach to include reader-viewers who have encountered other forms of suffering. Matesa claims that Byram's work with Brodsky conveys a message of "simple strength": "In that way, this project is less about breast cancer, being sick, and dying than it is about life—its impulses, joys, and difficulties, and the human struggle to experience these states fully in the ever-changing window frame of the present moment" (121). A practitioner of Buddhism, Byram advocates stillness, silence, and meditation as therapeutic strategies for herself as a cancer patient and as a narrative approach for reader-viewers who witness Brodsky's photographs. Near the end of her essay Matesa summarizes well the goals of *Knowing Stephanie.*

The photo-documentary, then, is not only for breast cancer patients; it is for anyone seeking a willingness to live fully, openly, and with rigorous honesty. Submitting to the lens on a regular basis helped Stephanie achieve a high level of openness about her life and its changes. If, as Brodsky suggests, the photograph enables the viewer to "feel for the complexity and difficulty of life," and so to be taken "somewhere else," then certainly this was true for Stephanie herself—the second viewer, after Brodsky, of each of these images. And it can be true, in turn, for each viewer, whether a breast cancer patient or not. (125)

Byram's sober reflections on living and dying meditatively contrast with Dina Rabinovitch's breezy tone in a blog posting of October 23, 2007, on "Take Off Your Running Shoes." This blog, which appeared a week before her death, featured a jaunty gray chapeau with feathers, a hat she deemed perfect for a wheelchair-bound patient on a public outing—because it looked stylish, concealed hair loss, and would not blow off, retrieval being impossible for a woman of limited mobility. "Many things I figured would be different in a wheelchair," the blog began.

> People making a particular effort not to talk over my head; being just the right height to press the Wait button on the traffic lights and so on, but one wheelchair effect I missed out, namely that I wear a hat to synagogue and when I lean my head back to look out from under the brim at people desperately trying to include me in conversations, well, that perfectly fine-fitting hat (previously) now goes sliding right off the back of my head. (www.dinablog.com)

A modified fedora designed by Pamela Savery solved the problem as "the perfectly chic, perfectly on-trend colour for the season, which is also cut close enough to the scalp to disguise newly falling hair and not slip off mid-gossip." This blog and the accompanying photograph elicited 116 reader comments within a week, initially fashion-oriented affirmations such as "What a totally FABULOUS hat!" and "You give Anna Wintour a run for her money in the style stakes . . . fantastic!" When news that Rabinovitch had died appeared on October 30, however, sartorial responses shifted to expressions of grief. "Such deep sorrow," wrote blogger Sonia Catan; "I grew to love and admire Dina so deeply, and her beautiful brave family travelling a road no one wants to have to travel. Valle Dina" (www.dinablog.com). "Terrible news," responded another blogger; "A wonderful woman, generous and alive at what must have been her most exhausted and despairing time. This marvelous hat—her last post—is a good expression of that vitality. Thank you, Dina. Though our loss cannot begin to compare with that of her family we will all—her virtual friends as well as those who knew her—miss her so very much. This comes with love, grief, and admiration" (www.dinablog.com). The authors of these and similar eulogies mourned Rabinovitch's death and positioned the photograph of her hat as communal memorial iconography.

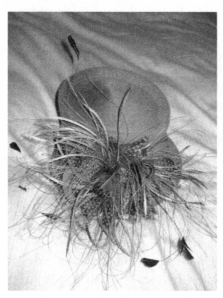

Dina Rabinovitch's hat. From her blog "Take Off Your Running Shoes." Courtesy of Anthony Julius.

As discussed in chapter 6, Annie Leibovitz's *A Photographer's Life* pays visual and narrative homage to her friend and partner Susan Sontag in indexical photographs of her living and dying breast cancer body. However, Leibovitz also memorializes Sontag in referential yet iconic photographs of her abandoned possessions, empty domestic spaces, and spectral silhouette. A photograph captioned *Susan's Shell Collection, King Street Sunporch, New York, 1990,* which follows the book's acknowledgment page, bears mute witness to the collector's travels to beaches where conch, starfish, and mussels conceal biologically simple life forms in aesthetically complex protective coverings. In this regard the shells function as a synecdoche for the absent body but enduring spirit of the woman who chose and arranged them. Another Leibovitz photograph from 1990, *Notes for The Volcano Lover, Berlin, 1990,* depicts tantalizing fragments of Sontag's handwritten manuscript covered with floating impenetrable phrases—"prologuette #3," "protection offered the city by the punctual liquefaction of a lump of its patron saint," "could Catherine be brought to top of mountain?"—words that pulse from the pages of Leibovitz's narrative and conjure the dead novelist as *unheimlich.* These enigmatic palimpsests, coupled with the image of an abandoned pencil that holds the papers down, create a visual collage that evokes reader melancholy and memorializes Sontag as a writer. A third photograph placed near the end of Leibovitz's memoir in photographs—a black-and-white cityscape of rooftops and balconies covered in snow, captioned *Looking Out from My Apartment to Susan's, London Terrace, New York, February 2005*—serves as a *memento mori* for the grieving photographer and for viewers aware that due to Sontag's death on December 28, 2004, her apartment was empty when the photo was taken. In the introduction to *A Photographer's Life* Leibovitz does not comment on these memorial images, but examined together they reflect the contours of her mourning and offer powerful traces of Sontag as traveler, collector, writer, New Yorker, lover.

Leibovitz does discuss the memorializing capacities of an arguably postindexical photograph captioned *Susan Sontag, Petra, Jordan, 1994,* the first image that viewers encounter in *A Photographer's Life* and a photograph now housed at the Metropolitan Museum of Modern Art (www.metmuseum.org/collections/search-the-collections/190040951). Sontag's slight silhouette assumes a spectral form in juxtaposition to the massive dark caverns through whose opening cleft an ornate white marble façade is visible. The photographer explains that she discovered this image in a shoebox while working on a memorial book to distribute to friends after Sontag's death.

> Photographs take on new meanings after someone dies. When I made the picture, I wanted her figure to give a sense of scale to the scene. But now I think of it as reflecting how much the world beckoned Susan. . . . Petra is an ancient city in southern Jordan that was more or less deserted for over a thousand years. . . . It's spectacular, with enormous columns and friezes. That's where Susan is standing. She loved art, architecture, history, travel, surprises. The photograph epitomizes all of that for me. . . . In retrospect, the photograph is also about the smallness of individual life. And since the façade is covered in funerary symbols, and since it was probably used as a tomb or a mausoleum, the picture sounds the themes of death and grief that wind through this book. (np)

Leibovitz's commentary acknowledges the photograph as a ghostly revenant that inscribes irretrievable loss, confronts relative human insignificance in the daunting sweep of history and time, and mourns its beloved subject's mortality, her adventurous life cut short by cancer as arbitrarily as the carvings of Petra were abandoned to lie in ruin.

Why might these images matter to audiences who did not know the dead women yet find themselves drawn to such elegiac representations? As Susanna Egan notes in *Mirror Talk,* photographs incorporated into autothanatography "open possibilities for grounding a viewer's experience in a life before and beyond the text" and raise awareness of "the subjectivity-in-representation of that life" (19). Such photographs facilitate collaborative construction of multiple subjectivities and anticipated mortalities, including those of photographer and viewer. Egan further argues that elegiac photographs and their accompanying written text "depend on the quondam presence of the subject and enact that presence by means of distinct but related codes," including an emotional confrontation with "instability in the living moment" (20).

Marianne Hirsch's discussion of the capacity of commemorative photographs to enter public spaces and "expand the postmemorial circle" further illuminates any effort to comprehend the elegiac authority of autothanatographic breast cancer photography. Drawing on Roland Barthes's theory in *Camera Lucida* regarding the *punctum,* that visual sensation evoked in viewers as a sudden jolt or wound, Hirsch in *Family Frames* affirms Barthes's contention that "by giving me the absolute past of the pose . . . the photograph tells me death in the future" (Barthes, 96, cited in Hirsch, 5). While she agrees with Barthes that photographs "possess an evidential force" that testifies to death's temporality, Hirsch notes his failure to acknowledge that "the structure of looking is reciprocal" and that photographer and viewer "collaborate on the reproduction of ideology": "Between the viewer and the recorded object, the viewer encounters, and/or projects, a screen made up of dominant mythologies and preconceptions that shapes the representation. Eye and screen are the very elements of ideology: our expectations circumscribe and determine what we show and what we see" (7). As instruments of ideology the camera, the photographer's gaze, the viewer's look, and the photographic text or exhibition have the potential to question, contest, or resist dominant interpretive ideologies, especially when the photographs under consideration encode trauma in narrative contexts.

When we consider "the moral dimensions of the instruments shaping our personal and cultural memory" (14), Hirsch continues, photography's capacity to evoke mourning becomes an essential topic to theorize: "Photographs, ghostly revenants, are very particular instruments of remembrance, since they are perched at the edge between memory and postmemory, and also, though differently, between memory and forgetting" (22). By *postmemory* Hirsh means not *beyond* memory but rather an intersubjective form of remembering that occurs through the "imaginative investment and creation" of witnesses once removed (22). When the closed circle of private photographs marking trauma and/or loss extends to include public viewers, power and grief circulate in new and multiple ways. Public displays of traumatic photographs thus constitute potential "spaces of connection between memory and postmemory," since viewers can mourn the untimely dead by confronting their visual traces (Hirsch, 247). Hirsch's theories can be applied to the photographic images of items left behind by Byram, Rabinovitch, and Sontag, images that arouse in many viewers an emotional solidarity that facilitates grieving and remembrance. Ulrich Baer makes a similar point in *Spectral Evidence: The Photography of Trauma* in claiming that viewers' imaginations can "invest the act of commemoration with ethical significance" through an "active, critical, and fundamentally creative stance" (155). If viewers witness traumatic or memorial images in private spaces, then grief and remembrance may remain individual, but if they/we witness such images in public exhibitions or venues, then mourning and remembering become communal.[5]

To conclude *Mammographies* I would like to call for a national memorial archive where literary works, unpublished manuscripts, photographs and photo-narratives, family scrapbooks, journals and diaries, DVDs and documentary films that chronicle the breast cancer experiences of women and men, whether famous or unknown, can be permanently housed.[6] Such an archive would provide space for public recognition, memorialization, and grieving for the dead alongside celebration of those "living in prognosis" (Jain, "Living in Prognosis," 77–78). I can also envision a public breast cancer project parallel to the AIDS memorial quilt (the Names Project), with its democratic gestures of shared grief and its capacity to raise consciousness about the HIV-AIDS pandemic.[7] AIDS does not recur, but breast cancer frequently does, often multiple times and in more virulent forms than that which originally manifested. This reality brings a sense of urgency to my call, as does the fact that worldwide breast cancer rates are rising rapidly; current projections posit that by 2020, 70 percent of all new cases will occur in developing countries (Kingsbury, 36). A U.S. breast cancer archive, along with a memorial quilt or a similar commemorative art project, would serve as a model for other locations and engage generations to come in public sites of remembrance and in collaborative acts of witness.

Appendix: Links to Selected Breast Cancer Websites and Blogs

Breast Cancer Advocacy Organizations and Websites

American Cancer Society, www.acs.org
The Assertive Cancer Patient, www.theassertivecancerpatient.org
Being Cancer Network, www.beingcancer.net
Breast Cancer Action, www.bcaction.org
The Breast Cancer Answers Project, www.canceranswers.org
The Breast Cancer Fund, www.breastcancerfund.org
Breast Cancer.Org , www.breastcancer.org
Breastlink, www.breastlink.org
Bright Pink, www.brightpink.org
Celebrate Life International, www.celebratelife.org
Community Breast Cancer, www.community.breast.cancer.org
Facing Our Risk of Cancer Empowered (FORCE), www.force.org
Living Beyond Breast Cancer, www.livingbeyondbreastcancer.org
National Breast Cancer Coalition, www.stopbreastcancer.org
Susan G. Komen for the Cure, www.komen.org
Y-Me National Breast Cancer Organization, www.y-me.org
Young Survival Coalition, www.youngsurvival.org

Selected Feminist Breast Cancer Blogs and Websites

Accidental Amazon, www.accidentalamazon.com
Boycott October, www.boycottoctober.com
Cancer Bitch, www.cancerbitch.com
Cancer Culture Chronicles, www.cancerculturenow.com
Chemobabe, www.chemobabe.com
Chemo Chicks, www.chemochicks.com
Fifty-Foot Blogger, www.thefifty-footblogger.com
Gayle Sulik, Pink Ribbon Blues, www.gaylesulik.com
Get Real About Breast Cancer, www.getrealaboutbreastcancer.com
Komenwatch, www.komenwatch.org

Peggy Orenstein, www.peggyorenstein.com
Planet Cancer, www.planetcancer.com
Ready, Pink, and Able, www.readypinkandable.com
Tania Katan, www.taniakatan.com
The SCAR Project, www.thescarproject.com

Notable BRCA and Previvor Blogs

BRCA Blues, www.brcablues.wordsmith.com
Boobs and Ovaries, www.boobnoophbrca1.blogspot.com
Breasts on My Chest, www.thebreastsonmychest.blogspot.com
Courage Is My Strength, www.courageismystrength.com
My BRCA Journey—PREVIVE!, www.goodbyebrcafate.blogspot.com
Positive Results, www.positiveresultsthebook.blogspot.com
Previvors Blog, www.previvors.com
Wearing My BRCA Genes, www.youngbrca1.wordpress.com
When the Genes Don't Fit, www.whenthegenesdontfit.blogspot.com
(See also FORCE and Bright Pink, above.)

Metastatic Breast Cancer Organizations and Websites

Advanced Breast Cancer, www.advancedbc.org
Advanced Breast Cancer Community, www.advancedbreastcancer
    community.org
BC Mets, www.bemets.org
Cancer Diaries, www.cancerby2.wordpress.com
Metastatic Breast Cancer Network, www.mbnc.org
METAvivor, www.metavivor.org

Notes

Introduction

1. According to the American Cancer Society and Susan G. Komen for the Cure, 226,870 new U.S. cases of invasive breast cancer and 63,300 cases of noninvasive (in situ) are estimated for 2012, and 39,500 will die of this disease; see www.cancer.org/ Cancer/Breastcancer/Detailed Guide/breast-cancer-key-statistics.html and www .komen.org/breastcancer/statistics.html.

2. For analysis of the global dimensions of breast cancer and elaboration of this statistic, see Kingsbury, 36–43.

3. See Davies and White, and also Lerner, 276–79, for the story of how King and her team at Berkeley proved that a gene related to breast cancer existed on chromosome 17, how Mark Skolnick and his colleagues at Myriad Genetics isolated the BRCA1 gene, and how BRCA2 was isolated. Deleterious mutations in either gene can be passed on to offspring by a carrier parent, and each child has a 50 percent chance of inheriting it. The term *previvor* originated with Sue Friedman, founder of the organization FORCE (Facing Our Risk of Cancer Empowered), which educates and supports women at risk for inheriting breast and ovarian cancer; see www.facingourrisk.org.

4. If a female infant inherits a BRCA mutation, estimates suggest that she will have a lifetime breast cancer risk of 85 percent (as opposed to 12 percent in the general U.S. population) and an ovarian cancer risk of up to 50 percent—hence the increasing turn to prophylactic mastectomy and oophorectomy by previvors. On this point, see www .facingourrisk.org and Gessen, 5–8. For evaluation of the efficacy of prophylactic mastectomy for high-risk women, see Hartmann; on patient satisfaction, see Brandberg et al. and Hallowell.

5. The SCAR Project exhibition began in Brooklyn in 2010. David Jay's photographs were exhibited in Cincinnati during September–October 2011 at Art Design Consultants and in New York at Openhouse Gallery in November 2011, in Washington, DC, in October 2012, and in Long Beach, January–February 2013. The film *Baring It All* premiered on PBS on July 9, 2011; for more information visit www.youtube.com/ watch?tv=G15w6Br5eZs and www.thescarproject.org.

6. To view images by Matuschka, see Ferraro and www.matuschka.com. For Spence's images, see Spence 1988 and 1995 or visit the Jo Spence Memorial Archive at www.hosted.aware.easynet.co.uk/jospence/ho1/htm. To view the iconic image of Metzger, visit www.deenametzger.com and click Tree.

7. For theoretical discussion of connections between autobiographical and photographic images, or "life writing" and "light writing," see Adams, Paul Jay, and Rugg.

8. Women of Ashkenazi Jewish descent have a 1 in 40 chance of testing positive for a BRCA mutation according to the American College of Obstetrics and Gynecology (www.acog.org); see also Gessen, 3–116. On the roles that race and ethnicity play

in breast cancer incidences and survival rates, see "The Color of Cancer," Kingsbury, LaTour, Patterson, Silver, and Williams.

9. See Ehrenreich, 43–50, for discussion of "pink kitsch" and culturally mandated cheerfulness in the face of cancer; see King, 101–15, for analysis of the "culture of survivorship and the tyranny of cheerfulness." For a history of the pink ribbon's use in breast cancer activism, see King, xii–xix; Ley, 118–22; McCormick, 44–46; and Sulik, 3–71.

10. For a *New York Times* article about the Komen controversy regarding Planned Parenthood funding, see Harris and Belluck. For an autobiographical account of founding Komen, see Brinker. For a trenchant critique of Komen's priorities, see Aschwanden. Another feminist blog that critiques Komen's perspective is that of S. L. Wisenberg, or "Cancer Bitch" (www.cancerbitch.blogspot.com), who features such 2012 postings as "News!!! Spine Discovered by Republican-founded Komen Foundation."

11. In "Living in Prognosis" Jain calls for an "elegiac politics" that recognizes identities for breast cancer patients other than that of survivor, "a space that allows for the agency and material humanity of suffering and death" (505). For a meditative study of the human effects of pain, see Thernstrom.

Chapter 1

1. More than 99 percent of breast cancers occur in women and less than 1 percent in men according to the Susan G. Komen for the Cure website (www.komen.org/breastcancer/statistics.html). An estimated 226,870 new cases of invasive breast cancer occurred in the United States during 2012, fewer than 1,500 of them in men. The vast majority of breast cancer memoirs have thus been written by women, but for a man's account, see Willis. This disease is also gendered due to the pervasive cultural fetishizing of women's breasts; on this point see Eisenstein, 69–70; Garland-Thomson, "Politics of Staring," 70–72; Olson, 110–20; and Yalom, 49–90.

2. King defines the breast cancer continuum as a trajectory that includes "risk, incidence, screening, diagnosis, treatment, survival, and mortality" (xviii). Regarding mammography as a breast imaging technology, McCormick notes that as of 2003 there were 8,600 mammography facilities in the United States, that a digital mammography machine typically costs $350,000 ($100,000 for analog), that 74.6 percent of U.S. women over forty had mammograms in 2005, and that although mammography continues to be widely viewed as the most viable and economical method of breast cancer detection available in the global North, the number of deaths prevented through the use of this technology has not changed during the past forty years. She discusses as well the Mammography Quality Standards Act of 1992, which required U.S. facilities to regulate standards more tightly than ever before (14–22). See Kingsbury for discussion of the paucity of screening technologies available to women in the global South.

3. Rugg explains the dual role of photographs in autobiographical narratives: "The presence of photographs in autobiography cuts two ways: it offers a visualization of the de-centered, culturally constructed self; and it asserts the presence of a living body through the power of photographic referentiality" (19). In addition, photographs in autobiographies "cue the reader into a complex play of signifiers that indicates the presence of a player, a person, upon whom text and images rebound" (21). See also Bal,

who notes that contemporary scholars of photography view it as "a form of writing, etymologically speaking 'with light'" and thus as beyond "the word-image opposition as it has been classically construed" (1). Bal further comments on the term *subject* as "bizarrely ambiguous" in that it "refers to the 'maker' . . . as well as the represented object" and offers a cautionary tale relevant to matters of ethical viewing that I take up later in this chapter: "That ambiguity harbours a truth about our relationship to the objects of analysis that warrants further scrutiny. It suggests that subject and object are conflated whenever we place ourselves, as observers, in the position of the maker" (6–7).

4. For discussion of photography as technology, see Barthes and Benjamin. For discussions of mammography as a screening technology for breast cancer, see Lerner; Ley, 22–23; McCormick, 14–22; and Olson, 131–32, 201–2. For analysis of the ways that breast cancer bodies are technologically mediated, see Ley, 182–96; McCormick, 87–146; Proctor, 255–56; and Stacey, 1–5.

5. My own previous work also addresses issues of illness, narrative, and embodiment; see DeShazer, 11–51.

6. For other feminist theorizations of chemo-related baldness, see Schultz and Sedgwick, "My Bald Head."

7. For a history of the pink ribbon's use in breast cancer activism, see King, xii–xix; Ley, 118–22; McCormick, 44–46; and Sulik, 3–71.

8. For assessments of the primacy of the face in early photography and in modern critical discourses on photographic portraiture, see Bal, 4–5, and Benjamin, 225–26.

9. Chapter 2 of this study addresses more extensively the issue of environmental silencing; see also Accad; Devra Davis; Eisenstein; Jain, "Cancer Butch"; Ley; McCormick; and Steingraber.

10. For additional information about Matuschka and her work, visit www.matuschka.com or www.songster.net/projects/matuschka; see also Matuschka, "The Body Beautiful"; Cartwright, 126–31; Dykstra; Van Schaick; and chapter 5 of this study.

Chapter 2

1. Ehrenreich's 2001 essay offers a trenchant critique of mainstream breast cancer culture from a feminist environmental perspective. For critical analysis of "White Glasses," see DeShazer, 237–42; Diedrich, 43–48; and Jain, "Cancer Butch," 504–6. Sedgwick also theorized breast cancer in *A Dialogue on Love* (1999). She died of this disease in 2009 at fifty-eight; see obituaries at www.nytimes.org and www.timesonline.co.uk. Herndl's own work as a theorist of breast cancer also deserves note; see "Reconstructing the Posthuman Feminist Body . . ." (2002).

2. On this point see Lerner, 276–90; McCormick; and chapter 3 of this study.

3. For additional discussion of ICI (Astra-Zeneca's) production of both tamoxifen and carcinogens, see Lerner, chapters 11 and 12; Ley, 38, 121–22; King, xx–xxi, 81–82; and McCormick, 37–38, 64–65. For a positive view of tamoxifen as a breast cancer treatment protocol, see Mukherjee, 216–22, 456–65.

4. On carcinogens that enter the body through mammary glands, see Devra Davis, 238–39, 288; McCormick, 128–29; "The Facts"; and Steingraber. Breast Cancer Action

and other environmentally focused breast cancer activist organizations cite 2011 studies that link the chemical Biphenyl-A (BPA) to breast cancer; on this point see Bader.

5. See Steingraber; Devra Davis, 338–61; and McCormick, 82–83, 91–100, for analysis of cancer alleys, environmental racism, and breast cancer mapping studies. For discussion of high breast cancer incidence rates among African Americans and Latinas in the Bay Area, see Klawiter, who reports that according to the Bay Area Partnership Latinas had the highest 1997 incident rate in the state of California, while African Americans had the second highest (154–56). See also Ley, who notes that according to WomenCare of Santa Cruz, Spanish-speaking women in the Watsonville, CA, area who contracted breast cancer were especially at risk because they lacked access to medical treatment and cancer support and services (20).

6. Lerner and Proctor recount this history in detail.

7. See Devra Davis, 281–84, for further articulation of estrogen-related claims, especially as relevant to young African American women's breast cancer risks. On the roles that race and ethnicity play more generally with regard to breast cancer risk, see "The Color of Cancer," LaTour, Silver, Kingsbury, and the essays in Williams.

8. For a summary of the results of the NIH's 2008 study of the health risks and benefits of hormone replacement therapy (HRT), see Heiss et al. This randomized U.S. trial ended early in 2005 when it became clear that HRT could lead to increased risk for breast cancer.

9. For more on automobile companies' participation in breast cancer cause-marketing, see King, vii–xxii, 13–15.

10. For an analysis of the relevance of Carson's environmental writing to contemporary cancer movements, see DeShazer, 242–52; Leopold, 113–40; Olson, 226–30; Proctor, 36–46; and the website of the Silent Spring Institute: www.silentspring.org.

11. It is important to note that the history of breast cancer is also well populated by physicians who work valiantly to overcome this disease and treat patients with professionalism and empathy; for an overview of that history, see Leopold, Lerner, Mukherjee, and Proctor.

12. For an analysis of prosthesis from a disability studies perspective, see Mitchell and Snyder, 6–10.

13. For further discussion of the politics of reconstruction, see Herndl, "Reconstructing," whose stance on reconstruction also differs from Lorde's and Eisenstein's. On recent developments related to breast reconstruction and women's experience of it, see Cobb and Starr; Crompvoets, "Comfort, Control, or Conformity" and "Prosthetic Fantasies"; "Progress and Promise," 28–30; and Singer. As Cobb and Starr note, it is difficult to access accurate statistics on the percentages of women who choose reconstruction during or after mastectomy; they cite one 2010 study that 25 percent of breast cancer patients do so but claim that anecdotal evidence provided in 2011 by surgical oncologists and plastic surgeons suggests that as many as 60 percent of U.S. women who require mastectomy undergo reconstructive surgery (99, fn 14).

14. For a related assessment of bodily hybridity following breast cancer treatment, see Herndl, "Reconstructing."

15. For thoughtful analyses of postmillennial directions in U.S. and transnational feminist breast cancer activism, see Ley, who discusses the shift "from pink to green,"

and Klawiter, who chronicles changing social movements and "cultures of activism."

16. For analysis of productive links between HIV/AIDS and breast cancer activism, see Boehmer, 26–39, 102–3, 137–45, and Cvetkovich, 156–238.

Chapter 3

1. See Boesky, Gabriel, Gessen, Port, and FORCE (www.facingourrisk.org) for additional narratives of prophylactic mastectomy. Both Boesky and Gabriel chronicle the impact of the BRCA gene on their lives and on the mother-daughter dynamic; Gabriel writes also about maternal abandonment and loss. As an investigative medical journalist with a BRCA mutation, Gessen interviews genetic counselors, oncologists, cancer researchers, and previvors and details her own decision-making process regarding prophylactic surgery. Port offers narratives of five high-risk women under forty who support one another in choosing prophylactic mastectomy. FORCE is the premier U.S. organization that raises awareness about previvor issues. See Gessen and Wexler for discussions of research into genetic risk and disease inheritance; see Couser, *Vulnerable Subjects,* for an analysis of the ethical considerations of seeking and acting on genetic information.

2. For an argument that genetic research should proceed with caution, see Hubbard and Wald. For a 2011 journalistic report on the disappointing results of once-promising targeted gene therapies, see Kolata.

3. For an assessment of the efficacy of prophylactic mastectomy in women with a family history of breast cancer, see Hartmann et al.

4. For an account of the research that led to the isolation of the BRCA genes, see Davies and White.

5. The statistic of a 1 in 40 chance of testing positive for BRCA1 or BRCA2 if one is of Ashkenazi Jewish descent comes from the American College of Obstetricians and Gynecologists (www.acog.org.).

6. For a different perspective on patient satisfaction after prophylactic mastectomy, see Hallowell.

7. Results of a 2008 study of quality of life for women after prophylactic mastectomy appear in Brandberg et al.

8. For critiques of triumphalist rhetoric in breast cancer culture, see Conway, 17–40; Ehrenreich; and chapter 5 of this study.

9. Ley discusses biomedical and biogenetic approaches to breast cancer causation as a "limited paradigm" that mistakenly emphasizes "reproductive, behavioral, clinical, and genetic factors over environmental factors" (4–6). See Ley, 77–121, 188, for an analysis of the successes of the U.S. feminist environmental breast cancer movement in bringing national attention to body burden studies that link chemical levels in the body to specific disease outcomes, in advocating a "precautionary principle" approach to the corporate development and commercial distribution of cancer-causing carcinogens, and in supporting the establishment of Breast Cancer and Environmental Research Centers at Michigan State University, the University of California at San Francisco, the University of Cincinnati, and Fox Chase Cancer Center in Philadelphia.

Chapter 4

1. To view illness photographs by/of Spence, see www.google.com/search?q=jo+sp ence+photography&hl; to see images of Wilke's "Intra-Venus," enter www.google.com/ search?q=hannah+wilke+intra+venus&hl.

2. See Prijatel for a layperson's analysis of current medical research on "chemo brain."

3. For a Bakhtinian theorization of the comic grotesque, see Stott, 87–91; for a Bakhtinian analysis of carnivalesque humor employed by hospital personnel and medical practitioners, see Gabbert and Salud.

4. For information about the Lance Armstrong Foundation, Armstrong's own experience of cancer, and his cancer awareness advocacy, visit www.livestrong.org.

5. For additional examples of cancer comics, see Andres; Batiuk; Bechdel; Fies; Marchetto; and Pekar and Brabner. For feminist theorizing of the postmillennial rise of graphic novels by women, see Chute.

6. To view the first twelve frames of *A Potpourri of Scans* see Block, "Miriam Engelberg, Cartoonist Who Chronicled Cancer," www.npr.org/templates/story/story .php?storyId=6303890.

7. For discussions of Susan G. Komen for the Cure's corporate politics and the breast cancer philanthropy of Avon, see Sulik; King, xix–xxx, 6–51; and Ley, 125–31.

8. Saranne Rothenberg, founder of ComedyCures, was diagnosed in 1999 with stage-four breast cancer and "made a vow to laugh at least 100 times a day." She subsequently began a career as a motivational speaker and hosted a "laugh line" telephone service—1-888-HA-HA-HA-HA—that in 2006 reached 4,000 people each month; see also Entemann.

Chapter 5

1. For more information on Matuschka's life and work, see her "The Body Beautiful"; Cartwright, 126–31; Dykstra; and Van Schaick. To view Matuschka's photographs, visit www.matuschka.com.

2. To view the photograph of Metzger by Hammid, visit www.deenametzger.com and click on Tree.

3. For further discussion of Metzger and this photograph's feminist history, see Cartwright, Dykstra, and van Schaick.

4. For more information on Spence's life and work, see *Cultural Sniping* and *Putting Myself in the Picture;* for theorization of her photographs, see Dykstra and van Schaick. To view Spence's photographs, visit the Jo Spence Memorial Archive at www .hosted.aware.easynet.co.uk/jospence/jo1/htm.

5. See Clark and Redgrave, Jay, and the introduction to this study for other examples of collaborative breast cancer photo-documentaries.

6. Other images from *Winged Victory* can be viewed at www.canceranswers.org/ gallery/myers.htm.

7. It is interesting to consider Myers's use of exotic, romantic, and sentimental images and discourses in *Winged Victory* in light of Rosemarie Garland-Thomson's

critique of "four primary visual rhetorics of disability" in contemporary culture: "the wondrous, the sentimental, the exotic, and the realistic" ("Politics of Staring," 58–72). While all four forms of visual rhetoric appear in Myers's collection, the first three forms (and from her perspective the most ethically problematic) are especially prominent.

8. See Conway, 17–39, 134–37, and Ehrenreich, 52–53, for additional critiques of triumphant discourses in breast cancer culture.

9. For discussion of twenty-first-century reconstruction options and the choices women are making, see Crompvoets, "Prosthetic Fantasies"; Erickson, Herndl, "Reconstructing"; "Progress and Promise," 28–30; and Singer. On the difficulty of getting accurate statistics regarding the number of U.S. women who choose breast reconstruction after mastectomy, see Cobb and Starr, 99, fn. 14.

10. My June 2, 2012, Google search for breast cancer tattoos produced an astonishing 1,590,000 results. For analysis of this phenomenon, visit www.1st-in-breastcancer.com/breast-cancer-tattoos-for-women. To view additional breast tattoos, visit www.youtube.com/watch?v=dkvLytqhAc. Not all breast cancer tattoos appear on patients' post-mastectomy chests; many constitute activist gestures of solidarity; see www.pinterest.com/facecancer2gthr/inspired-ink-cancer-tattoos for a range of cancer-related tattoos on various parts of the subjects' bodies.

11. To view several images from *Heroines,* visit www.events.mnhs.org/media/news/release.cfm?ID=837.

12. Information and several images from *Caring for Cynthia* can be found at www.caringforcynthia.com.

13. On matters of photographic temporality, see Avrahami, 97–98; Barthes, 13–15, 97–99; and Sontag, *On Photography,* 17–18.

14. On the ontological significations of photographs, see Sontag, *On Photography,* 23–24.

15. Brodsky and Byram discussed their collaboration in a 1994 interview with David Demerest; see "At Charlee's House." They also collaborated on an Emmy-award-winning documentary film, *Stephanie,* produced by Mary Rawson and shown nationally on PBS in October 2000.

16. In *Vulnerable Subjects* Couser advocates "principalism" as a guideline for evaluating biographical or visual representations of vulnerable subjects, defined as "respect for autonomy, beneficence, and justice" (preface).

17. Personal email from Brodsky to author, June 5, 2012.

Chapter 6

1. In a posthumously published journal entry from 1977 Sontag described *Illness as Metaphor* as "an attempt to 'do' literary criticism in a new way but for a pre-modern purpose: to criticize the world" and claimed that study was "about how the metaphoric understanding, and the moralization of a disease, belies the medical realities" (*As Consciousness,* 453–54). For an analysis of the importance of *Illness as Metaphor* to feminist theories of illness and embodiment, see DeShazer, 11–18, and Diedrich, 26–32.

2. See, however, Sontag, *As Consciousness,* which covers the period when she was treated for breast cancer and features occasional commentary on her illness and

her confrontation with mortality. On page 401, for example, she describes humans "in youth, growing up, floated up by-with-the body; ageing or sick, the body drifting downwards, sinking or plummeting, leaving the self stranded, evaporating," and on page 401 she refers wryly to "my cancer minstrel show."

3. Prior to its exhibitions in London and Europe, *A Photographer's Life* was exhibited at the Brooklyn Museum, The Corcoran Gallery in Washington, DC, the Legion of Honor Museum in San Francisco, and the Fox Theater in Atlanta. I saw the exhibition at the National Portrait Gallery in London, February 1, 2009. The term *American Master* comes from a PBS series by that title that in 2008 featured a documentary film about Leibovitz directed by her sister, Barbara Leibovitz.

4. On this point see Henderson, "Access and Consent in Public Photography," 276.

5. Based on his interview with Leibovitz, Guthmann explains her decision to exhibit and publish these images as follows: "The decision to include the shots of Sontag hospitalized, dying, and then deceased were made, she says, after enormous deliberation. Leibovitz consulted with Sontag's sister, Judith Cohen, and her agent, Andrew Wylie, co-executor of Sontag's estate ('I wanted to make sure everyone was comfortable'), but not Sontag's son, David Rieff. 'I don't talk to David,' she said with a sad, resigned frown. 'Everyone deals with death in a different way, and it didn't end well with David.'"

6. The bathtub images of Sontag from *My Apartment in London Terrace* can be viewed at www.ganasdeananas.tumblr.com. Other widely circulating post-mastectomy photographs include Hella Hammid's portrait of poet Deena Metzger's tattooed mastectomy scar, sold as a poster in the late 1970s and reproduced in the 1992 edition of Metzger's *Tree* (www.deenametzger.com); the model Matuschka's self-portrait of her draped, flat chest on the cover of the *New York Times Magazine* in 1993, which accompanied an article by Susan Ferraro, "The Anguished Politics of Breast Cancer"; and the photographic depictions of women's post-surgical breasts in Amelia Davis, Myers, and Nikpay, as discussed in chapter 5 of this study. For additional information about Matuschka's breast cancer photographs, see www.matuschka.com; www.songster.net/projects/matuschka; Cartwright, 126–31; Dykstra; and Van Schaick.

7. "Leaving Seattle, November 15, 2004" can be viewed at www.flickr.com; the contact sheet images of Sontag in the funeral home can be viewed at www.bagnewsnotes.typepad.com/misc/leibovitz-sontag-deceased.jpg.

8. For further discussion of photographs depicting trauma, see Baer; Butler, *Frames of War*; Hirsch; and Pollock. For analysis of the perils of portraiture in a post-traumatic age, see Bal and Saltzman.

9. With regard to the history of photographing the dead as a form of *memento mori*, see Gilbert, 222–41, and Hirsch, 5–23, 245–47.

10. In "Mourning and Melancholia" Freud describes the work of mourning as a "testing of reality" necessary to prove that "the loved object no longer exists," an effort of detachment that initiates an emotional struggle in the bereaved to be "carried through bit by bit, under great expense of time and cathectic energy, while all the time the existence of the lost object is continued in the mind" (165–66). This description sheds light on Rieff's account as he probes his response to his mother's final illness and death.

11. For further discussion of Rieff's writing process and ethical decisions, see Horton.

12. Reviewers who argue that Leibovitz exploits Sontag include Karnasiewicz, McRobbie, Thomson, and Roberta Smith.

13. For discussion of Hirsch's views on expanding the "postmemorial circle," see my Afterword.

14. These statistics come from "The Facts and Nothing but the Facts," Breast Cancer Action, http://www.bcaction.org/index.php?page=facts.

15. See Nancy K. Miller for a different conclusion, however. In her analysis of Sontag's "posthumous life" as revealed in Leibovitz's photographs, in obituaries, and in Rieff's memoir, Miller agrees with Rieff that Leibovitz's memorialization is ethically problematic. She speculates that Sontag, who wrote about photography as invasive and appropriative, would not have sanctioned the publication of photographs of herself dying or dead.

16. See Pollock, "Femininity," for an extended critical analysis of Ettinger's art and further theorization of the matrixial gaze.

17. In his analysis of viewers' relationships to traumatic photographs Baer considers how our imaginations can "invest the act of commemoration with ethical significance" through an "active, critical, and fundamentally creative stance" (155). On ethical representations of victims of war and/or torture, see also Sontag, "Regarding the Torture of Others," and Butler, *Frames of War,* 63–100.

18. In "Cancer Butch" Jain probes the corporate underpinnings of U.S. breast cancer awareness and activism and advocates as a progressive response an "elegiac politics": "Rather than a call to action, an elegiac politics recognizes the basic human costs of U.S. capitalism." Jain attributes the phrase *elegiac politics* to AIDS activist Derek Simons. See also Jain, "Living in Prognosis," 77–92, and chapter 2 of this study, which analyzes Jain's theories in detail.

19. The comments cited in regard to Rieff's work are those of reviewers Roiphe (11), Sacks (as quoted on the book jacket of *Swimming in a Sea of Death*), and Johnson and Murray (np). The comments cited in regard to Leibovitz's book and/or photographic exhibition are those of reviewers Roberta Smith, Karnasiewicz, and Thomson. Obviously aesthetic as well as ethical judgments inform reviews of Rieff's and Leibovitz's work, and graphic photographs of cancer may offend audiences more than graphic words describing it do. Still, it disturbs me that Sontag's lover received much condemnation for an intimate public representation parallel to that for which her son received mostly accolades; on this point, see McKinney, who suggests that Leibovitz's photographs of Sontag upset some viewers because they represent "an ethics of queer domesticity." To be sure, a few reviewers lauded Leibovitz's photographs of Sontag as courageous; see Garwood, Guthmann, and Wilson. I also found two reviewers who objected on ethical grounds to Rieff's representation of his mother's death in his memoir, Mars-Jones and Zuger.

Chapter 7

1. See Adams and Rugg for further theorization of this point.

2. See Brodsky and Byram, Butler and Rosenblum, Lynch and Richards, Middle-brook, and Romm for other examples of cancer autothanatography. For further analysis of this genre, see Egan, DeShazer, 223–37, and chapter 5 of this study.

3. For further consideration of cultural assumptions about maternal transcendence, see Rich, chapter 7.

4. See Couser, *Vulnerable Subjects,* for further discussion of ethical representation of the dead, dying, and/or severely disabled.

5. Despite the fact that Ruth Picardie's narrative does not discuss the feminist breast cancer movement, it is important to note that Ruth's sister Justine Picardie and Beth Wagstaff launched a U.K. breast cancer organization, the Lavender Trust, shortly after Ruth's death and in her honor. Its mission is to provide information and support to young women with this disease. Part of the proceeds from sales of *Before I Say Goodbye* went to this organization, and Picardie's family has continued involvement; see www.lavendertrust.org.uk.

6. For further discussion of illness as infantilizing, see Ehrenreich and Stacey, 1–5.

7. For feminist perspectives on breast cancer experimental drug trials, see Ley and McCormick. For a medical doctor's perspective on targeted therapies for breast cancer, see Mukherjee, 413–22.

8. For more on class-related issues regarding access to breast cancer treatment, see Devra Davis and Eisenstein.

9. See Phelan for a compelling theorization of grief and mourning in the context of the AIDS pandemic.

10. To the best of my knowledge no U.S. breast cancer organizations have floated the idea of a memorial quilt, but I consider it a project worth exploring. On the relevance of HIV/AIDS activism to breast cancer activism, see Boehmer and Jain, "Cancer Butch," 527–28. For information on the AIDS memorial quilt, see Cvetkovich, 156–238; Morris, 190–246; and wwwaidsquilt.org.

Afterword

1. For analysis of Lin's *Vietnam Veterans Memorial* project, see Saltzman, 7–12, and Mitchell, 379–81.

2. For discussion of the ethical implications and public impact of *Bunker Hill Monument Project,* see Saltzman, 28–47. For an analysis of Boltanski's public art projects, see Saltzman, 14, 92–93, and Hirsch, 260–63. The full title of Walker's *Gone* is *Gone, An Historical Romance of a Civil War as It Occurred Between the Dusky Thighs of One Young Negress and Her Heart;* see Saltzman, 58–69, for an analysis of this work's aesthetic strategies, memorializing capacities, and controversial status in the art world.

3. For further consideration of such memorial practices, see Gilbert's chapter "Millennial Mourning" in *Death's Door,* 242–92.

4. Brodsky and Byram discussed their collaboration in a 1994 interview with David Demerest; see "At Charlee's House."

5. Numerous exhibitions of breast cancer art have circulated in the United States and beyond in recent years, including the Art.Rage.Us exhibitions from San Francisco to New Orleans to Hong Kong during the late 1990s and early twenty-first century; see Kenneth Baker and www.tulane.edu/~newcomb/artrage.html. There have also been many decorative bra exhibitions such as *Cups Full of Hope* in 2010 in Washington, DC,

and *Dance of Life: Bras for Breast Cancer* in 2010 in Dallas; see www.washingtonpost. com/wp-syn/content/article as well as www.web.me.com/juneannepack/BRAS_For_ Breast_Cancer. Bra exhibitions have extended as far as Brazil. A 2010 São Paolo exhibition was entitled *The Bra: The Battle Continues—Campaign against Breast Cancer;* for information about the artists and goals of this project, see www.nydailynews.com/ entertainment/music/galleries/bras_for_a_cause. An exhibition entitled *Voices and Visions: Standing on the Bridge between Health and Disease,* which features breast cancer art in many mediums, was on display during June 2011 in Portland, Oregon, and traveled nationally through 2012; see www.carenhelenerudman.com. And a 2010 *Pink Lady Art Show* in Australia raised money for Breast Cancer Network Australia and the National Breast Cancer Foundation; see www.pinkladyart.com.au. Additional paintings related to breast cancer can be viewed at the website of The Breast Cancer Answers Project, www.canceranswers.org/gallery. My hope would be that art from such exhibitions could be housed in a national breast cancer archive alongside art that is overtly elegiac, resistant, and/or memorial in tone and scope.

6. A parallel project that could serve as a model is the national Lesbian Herstory Archive in Brooklyn, NY; see Cvetkovich, 78–79, 240–51, 269–70.

7. For more on the AIDS memorial quilt see Cvetkovich, 156–238; Gilbert, 288–90; Morris 190–246; and www.aidsquilt.org.

Works Cited

Accad, Evelyne. *The Wounded Breast: Intimate Journeys through Cancer.* Melbourne: Spinifex, 2001.

Adams, Timothy Dow. *Light Writing and Life Writing: Photography in Autobiography.* Chapel Hill: University of North Carolina Press, 2000.

Ahmed, Sara. *The Cultural Politics of Emotion.* New York: Routledge, 2004.

Andres, Kaylin Marie. "Cancer Is Hilarious: *Terminally Illin'*." http://cancerisnotfunny. blogspot.com.

Aschwanden, Christie. "The Real Scandal: Science Denialism at Susan G. Komen for the Cure." http://www.lastwordonnothing.com/2012/02/08/komen.

"At Charlee's House." David Demerest interview with Charlee Brodsky and Stephanie Byram. Aug. 8, 1994. http://cultronix.eserver.org/stephanie/interview.

Avrahami, Einat. *The Invading Body: Reading Illness Autobiographies.* Charlottesville: University of Virginia Press, 2007.

Bader, Eleanor J. "Snipping Pink Sentimentality: Persisting on the Whys of Breast Cancer." *On the Issues Magazine,* May 2011. www.ontheissuesmagazine. com/2011spring_Bader.php.

Baer, Ulrich. *Spectral Evidence: The Photography of Trauma.* Cambridge: MIT Press, 2002.

Baker, Gail Konop. *Cancer Is a Bitch: Or, I'd Rather Be Having a Midlife Crisis.* Cambridge, MA: Da Capo Press, 2008.

Baker, Kenneth. "Confronting Breast Cancer through Art: 'Art.Rage.Us' Show at Main Library." http://www.sfgate.com/1998-04-24/entertainment/17718053_1_breast.

Bakhtin, Mikhail. *Rabelais and His World.* Trans. Helene Iswolsky. Cambridge: MIT Press, 1984.

Bal, Mieke. "Light Writing: Portraiture in a Post-Traumatic Age." *Mosaic* 37, no. 4 (Dec. 2004): 1–19. http://proquest.umi.com/pdqweb?/index=0&sid=1&srchmod e=1&vinst=PROD&fmt=3&st.

Barthes, Roland. *Camera Lucida: Reflections on Photography.* Trans. Richard Howard. 1980. New York: Noonday Press, 1990.

Batiuk, Tom. *Lisa's Story/The Other Shoe.* Kent, OH: Kent State University Press, 2007.

Baudelaire, Charles. "On the Essence of Laughter, and, in General, on the Comic in the Plastic Arts." 1855. In *Selected Writings on Art and Artists,* ed. Robert Baldick and Betty Radice, trans. P. E. Charvet, 140–62. Middlesex: Penguin Books, 1972.

Bechdel, Alison. *The Essential Dykes to Watch Out For.* New York: Houghton Mifflin, 2008.

Benjamin, Walter. "The Work of Art in the Age of Mechanical Reproduction." *Illuminations: Essays and Reflections,* ed. Hannah Arendt, trans. Harry Zohn, 217–51. New York: Schocken Books, 1968.

Bennett, Mary Payne, and Cecile Lengacher. "Humor and Laughter May Influence

Health II: Complementary Therapies and Humor in a Clinical Population." Oct. 30, 2008. http://www.pubmedcentral.nih.gov.

Bernard, Jami. "The Ha-Ha Sisterhood." *MAMM,* Dec. 2008–Jan. 2009. http://www.mamm.com/highlights.php?&9backid.

Bishop, Lauren. "SCAR Project Shows Raw Reality of Breast Cancer." *USA Today,* Sept. 30, 2011. http://www.usatoday.com/news/health/medical/breastcancer/story/2011-09-30/SCAR-Project-shows-raw-reality-of-breast-cancer-50616200/1.html.

Blackburn, Amy S. *Caring for Cynthia: A Caregiver's Journey through Breast Cancer.* San Rafael, CA: Verve Editions, 2008.

Block, Melissa. "Miriam Engelberg, Cartoonist Who Chronicled Cancer," Oct. 18, 2006. http://www.npr.org/templates/story/story.php?storyId=6303890.

Boehmer, Ulrike. *The Personal and the Political: Women's Activism in Response to the Breast Cancer and AIDS Epidemics.* New York: New York University Press, 2000.

Boesky, Amy. *What We Have: One Family's Inspiring Story about Love, Loss, and Survival.* New York: Penguin Books, 2010.

Brandberg, Y., et al. "Psychological Reactions, Quality of Life, and Body Image after Bilateral Prophylactic Mastectomy in Women at High Risk for Breast Cancer: A Prospective One-Year Follow-up Study." *Journal of Clinical Oncology* 26, no. 24 (Aug. 2008): 3943–49.

Brinker, Nancy G., with Joni Rodgers. *Promise Me: How a Sister's Love Launched the Global Movement to End Breast Cancer.* New York: Three Rivers Press, 2010.

Brodsky, Charlee, and Stephanie Byram. *Knowing Stephanie.* Pittsburgh: University of Pittsburgh Press, 2003.

Bronfen, Elisabeth M. *Over Her Dead Body: Death, Femininity, and the Aesthetic.* London: Routledge, 1992.

Bryan, Elizabeth. *Singing the Life: The Story of a Family in the Shadow of Cancer.* London: Vermillion, 2007.

Butler, Judith. *Frames of War: When Is Life Grievable?* London: Verso Books, 2009.

Butler, Judith. "Performative Acts and Gender Constitution: An Essay in Phenomenology and Feminist Theory." In *Performing Feminisms: Feminist Critical Theory and Theatre,* ed. Sue-Ellen Case, 270–82. Baltimore: Johns Hopkins University Press, 1990..

Butler, Judith. *Precarious Life: The Powers of Mourning and Violence.* London: Verso Books, 2004.

Butler, Sandra, and Barbara Rosenblum. *Cancer in Two Voices.* Duluth, MN: Spinsters Ink, 1991.

Carr, Kris. *Crazy Sexy Cancer Tips.* Guilford, CT: Globe Pequot Press, 2007.

Carson, Rachel. *Silent Spring.* 1962. Boston: Houghton Mifflin, 2002.

Cartwright, Lisa. "Community and the Public Body in Breast Cancer Media Activism." *Wild Science: Reading Feminism, Medicine and the Media,* ed. Janine Marchessault and Kim Sawchuk, 120–38. London: Routledge, 2000.

Chute, Hillary L. *Graphic Women: Life Narrative and Contemporary Comics.* New York: Columbia University Press, 2010.

Clark, Annabel, and Lynn Redgrave. *Journal: A Mother and Daughter's Recovery from Breast Cancer.* New York: Umbrage Editions, 2004.

Cobb, Shelley, and Susan Starr. "Breast Cancer, Breast Surgery, and the Makeover Metaphor." *Social Semiotics* 22, no. 1 (Feb. 2012): 83–102.

Cohen, Deborah A., and Robert M. Gelfand. *Just Get Me Through This! A Practical Guide to Coping with Breast Cancer.* 2nd ed. New York: Kensington Books, 2011.

"The Color of Cancer: The Role of Race and Ethnicity in Cancer." *CURE (Cancer Updates, Research and Education) Supplement.* Winter 2009.

Conway, Kathlyn. *Illness and the Limits of Expression.* Ann Arbor: University of Michigan Press, 2007.

Couser, G. Thomas. *Recovering Bodies: Illness, Disability, and Life Writing.* Madison: University of Wisconsin Press, 1997.

Couser, G. Thomas. *Vulnerable Subjects: Ethics and Life Writing.* Ithaca: Cornell University Press, 2004.

Crompvoets, Samantha. "Comfort, Control, or Conformity: Women Who Choose Breast Reconstruction Following Mastectomy." *Health Care for Women International* 27, no. 1 (2006): 75–93.

Crompvoets, Samantha. "Prosthetic Fantasies: Loss, Recovery, and the Marketing of Wholeness after Breast Cancer." *Social Semiotics* 22, no. 1 (Feb. 2012): 107–20.

Cvetkovich, Ann. *An Archive of Feeling: Trauma, Sexuality, and Lesbian Public Cultures.* Durham: Duke University Press, 2003.

Davies, Kevin, and Michael White. *Breakthrough: The Race to Find the Breast Cancer Gene.* New York: Macmillan, 1995.

Davis, Amelia. *The First Look.* Urbana: University of Illinois Press, 2000.

Davis, Devra. *The Secret History of the War on Cancer.* New York: Basic Books, 2007.

DeShazer, Mary K. *Fractured Borders: Reading Women's Cancer Literature.* Ann Arbor: University of Michigan Press, 2005.

Diedrich, Lisa. *Treatments: Language, Politics, and the Culture of Illness.* Minneapolis: University of Minnesota Press, 2007.

Dunnavant, Sylvia, ed. *Celebrating Life: African-American Women Speak Out about Breast Cancer.* Dallas: USFI, 1995.

Dykstra, Jean. "Putting Herself in the Picture: Autobiographical Images of Illness and the Body." *Afterimage,* Sept.–Oct. 1995. http://findarticles.com/p/articles/mi_m2479/is_n2_v23/ai_17789645.

Egan, Susanna. *Mirror Talk: Genres of Crisis in Contemporary Autobiography.* Chapel Hill: University of North Carolina Press, 1999.

Ehrenreich, Barbara. "Welcome to Cancerland." *Harper's Magazine,* November 2001, 43–53.

Eisenstein, Zillah. *Manmade Breast Cancers.* Ithaca: Cornell University Press, 2001.

Engelberg, Miriam. *Cancer Made Me a Shallower Person: A Memoir in Comics.* New York: HarperCollins, 2006.

Entemann, Dalene. "Comedy Cures." April 28, 2006. http://www.thecancerblog.com.

Ericksen, Julia A. *Taking Charge of Breast Cancer.* Berkeley: University of California Press, 2008.

Ettinger, Bracha L. *The Matrixial Borderspace.* Minneapolis: University of Minnesota Press, 2006.

"The Facts and Nothing But the Facts." Breast Cancer Action. April 24, 2009. http://www.bcaction.org/index.php?page=facts.

Ferraro, Susan. "The Anguished Politics of Breast Cancer." *New York Times Magazine,* Aug. 15, 1993, 24–27, 58–62.

Fies, Brian. *Mom's Cancer.* New York: Abrams Image, 2006.

Frank, Arthur W. *The Wounded Storyteller: Body, Illness, and Ethics.* Chicago: University of Chicago Press, 1995.

Freud, Sigmund. "Mourning and Melancholia." 1917. Trans. Joan Riviere. In *General Psychological Theory,* ed. and intro. Philip Rieff. New York: Collier, 1963.

Freud, Sigmund. "On Humour." 1927. In *The Standard Edition of the Complete Psychological Works of Sigmund Freud,* trans. and ed. James Strachey, 21:159–66. London: Hogarth Press, 1957.

Freud, Sigmund. "On Narcissism: An Introduction." 1914. In *The Standard Edition of the Complete Psychological Works of Sigmund Freud,* trans. and ed. James Strachey, 14:73–102. London: Hogarth Press, 1957.

Gabbert, Lisa, and Antonio Salud II. "On Slanderous Words and Bodies Out-of-Control: Hospital Humor and the Medical Carnivalsque." In *The Body in Medical Culture,* ed. Elizabeth Klaver, 209–27. Albany: SUNY Press, 2010.

Gabriel, Sarah. *Eating Pomegranates: A Memoir of Mothers, Daughters, and the BRCA Gene.* New York: Scribner, 2009.

Garland-Thomson, Rosemarie. "The Politics of Staring: Visual Rhetorics of Disability in Popular Photography." In *Disability Studies: Enabling the Humanities,* ed. Sharon L. Snyder et al., 56–75. New York: MLA Press, 2002.

Garland-Thomson, Rosemarie. *Staring: How We Look.* Oxford: Oxford University Press, 2009.

Garwood, Deborah. Review of "A Photographer's Life, 1990–2005," exhibition by Annie Leibovitz, Brooklyn Museum. *Artcritical.com,* Feb. 2007. http://www.artcritical.com/garwood/DGLeibovitz.htm.

Gessen, Masha. *Blood Matters: From Inherited Illness to Designer Bodies—How the World and I Found Ourselves in the Future of the Gene.* New York: Harcourt, 2009.

Gilbert, Sandra M. *Death's Door: Modern Dying and the Ways We Grieve.* New York: W. W. Norton, 2006.

Gilmore, Leigh. *The Limits of Autobiography: Trauma and Testimony.* Ithaca: Cornell University Press, 2001.

Guthmann, Edward. "Love, Family, Celebrity, Grief—Leibovitz Puts Her Life on Display in Photo Memoir." *San Francisco Chronicle,* Nov. 1, 2006. http://www.sfgate.com/cgi-bin/article.cgi?f=/c/a/2006/11/01/DDG/html.

Hallowell, Nina. "Reconstructing the Body or Reconstructing the Woman? Problems of Prophylactic Mastectomy for Hereditary Breast Cancer Risk." In *Ideologies of Breast Cancer: Feminist Perspectives,* ed. Laura K. Potts, 153–80. London: Macmillan Press, 2000.

Harris, Gardiner, and Pam Belluck. "Uproar as Breast Cancer Group Ends Partnership with Planned Parenthood." *New York Times,* Feb. 1, 2012. http://www.nytimes.com/2012/02/02/us/uproar-as-komen-foundation-cuts-money-to-planned-parenthood.html.

Hartmann, L. C., et al. "Efficacy of Bilateral Prophylactic Mastectomy in Women with a Family History of Breast Cancer." *New England Journal of Medicine* 340, no. 2 (Jan. 1999): 77–84.

Heiss, G., et al. "Health Risks and Benefits Three Years after Stopping Randomized Treatment with Estrogen and Progestin." *Journal of the American Medical Association* 299, no. 9 (March 2008): 1036–45.

Henderson, Lisa. "Access and Consent in Public Photography." *The Photography Reader,* ed. Liz Wells, 275–87. London: Routledge, 2003.

Herndl, Diane Price. "Our Breasts, Our Selves: Identity, Community, and Ethics in Cancer Autobiographies." *Signs: Journal of Women in Culture and Society* 32, no. 1 (Autumn 2006): 221–45.

Herndl, Diane Price. "Reconstructing the Posthuman Feminist Body Twenty Years after Audre Lorde's *Cancer Journals.*" In *Disability Studies: Enabling the Humanities,* ed. Sharon L. Snyder, Brenda Brueggemann, and Rosemarie Garland-Thomson, 144–55. New York: MLA Press, 2002.

Hirsch, Marianne. *Family Frames: Photography, Narrative, and Postmemory.* Cambridge: Harvard University Press, 1997.

Horton, Scott. "Six Questions for David Rieff, Author of 'Swimming in a Sea of Death.'" *Harper's Magazine,* Mar. 6, 2008. http:// www.harpers.org/archive/2008/03/ hbc90002558.

Hubbard, Ruth, and Elijah Wald. *Exploding the Gene Myth: How Genetic Information Is Produced and Manipulated by Scientists, Physicians, Employers, Insurance Companies, Educators, and Law Enforcers.* 2nd ed. Boston: Beacon Press, 1999.

Isaak, Jo Anna. "In Praise of Primary Narcissism: The Last Laughs of Jo Spence and Hannah Wilke." In *Interfaces: Women/Autobiography/Image/Performance,* ed. Sidonie Smith and Julia Watson, 49–68. Ann Arbor: University of Michigan Press, 2002.

Jain, S. Lochlann. "Be Prepared." In *Against Health: How Health Became the New Morality,* ed. Anna Kirkland and Jonathan Metzl, 170–82. New York: New York University Press, 2010.

Jain, S. Lochlann. "Cancer Butch." *Cultural Anthropology* 22, no. 4 (2007): 501–38.

Jain, S. Lochlann. "Living in Prognosis: Toward an Elegiac Politics." *Representations* 98 (Spring 2007): 77–92.

Jarvis, Debra. *It's Not about the Hair: and Other Certainties of Life and Cancer.* Seattle: Sasquatch Books, 2007.

Jay, David. *The SCAR Project: Breast Cancer Is Not a Pink Ribbon.* Vol. 1, 2011. http:// www.thescarproject.org.

Jay, Paul. "Posing: Autobiography and the Subject of Photography." In *Autobiography and Postmodernism,* ed. Kathleen Ashley, Leigh Gilmore, and Gerald Peters, 191–211. Amherst: University of Massachusetts Press, 1994.

Johnson, Diane, and John F. Murray. "Will to Live." Review of *Swimming in a Sea of Death: A Son's Memoir,* by David Rieff. *New York Review of Books* 55, no. 2 (Feb. 14, 2008). http://www.nybooks.com/articles/21010.

Karnasiewicz, Sarah. "Annie Leibovitz's Reckless Candor." *salon.com,* Nov. 18, 2006. http://www.salon.com/ent/feature/2006/11/18/leibovitz.

King, Samantha. *Pink Ribbons, Inc.: Breast Cancer and the Politics of Philanthropy.* Minneapolis: University of Minnesota Press, 2006.

Kingsbury, Kathleen. "The Changing Face of Breast Cancer." *Time,* Oct. 15, 2007, 36–43.

Klawiter, Maren. *The Biopolitics of Breast Cancer: Changing Cultures of Disease and Activism.* Minneapolis: University of Minnesota Press, 2008.

Klefsted, Ann. "Interview with Jila Nikpay." *10,000 Arts,* Oct. 29, 2007. www.mnartists.org/article.do?rid-164813.

Knopf-Newman, Marcy Jane. *Beyond Slash, Burn, and Poison: Transforming Breast Cancer Stories into Action.* New Brunswick: Rutgers University Press, 2004.

Kolata, Gina. "How Bright Promise in Cancer Testing Fell Apart." *New York Times,* July 8, 2011, A1, 14.

LaTour, Kathy. "The Many Shades of Survivorship." *CURE: Cancer Updates, Research and Education (Supplement),* Winter 2009, 27–31.

Leibovitz, Annie. Exhibition of works from *A Photographer's Life, 1990–2005.* London: National Portrait Gallery, Oct. 16, 2008–Feb. 1, 2009.

Leibovitz, Annie. *A Photographer's Life, 1990–2005.* New York: Random House, 2006.

Leibovitz, Barbara. *Annie Leibovitz: Life Through a Lens.* PBS American Masters Series, 2008. DVD.

Leopold, Ellen. *A Darker Ribbon: Breast Cancer, Women, and Their Doctors in the Twentieth Century.* Boston: Beacon, 1999.

Lerner, Barron H. *The Breast Cancer Wars: Fear, Hope, and the Pursuit of a Cure in Twentieth-Century America.* Oxford: Oxford University Press, 2001.

Lewis, Shelley. *Five Lessons I Didn't Learn from Cancer (And One Big One I Did).* New York: Penguin, 2008.

Ley, Barbara L. *From Pink to Green: Disease Prevention and the Environmental Breast Cancer Movement.* New Brunswick: Rutgers University Press, 2009.

Lord, Catherine. *The Summer of Her Baldness: A Cancer Improvisation.* Austin: University of Texas Press, 2004.

Lorde, Audre. *A Burst of Light.* Ithaca: Firebrand Books, 1988.

Lorde, Audre. *The Cancer Journals.* San Francisco: Spinsters Ink, 1980.

Lucas, Geralyn. *Why I Wore Lipstick to My Mastectomy.* New York: St. Martin's, 2004.

Lynch, Dorothea, and Eugene Richards. *Exploding into Life.* New York: Aperture, 1986.

Marchetto, Marisa Acocella. *Cancer Vixen.* New York: Alfred A. Knopf, 2006.

Mars-Jones, Adam. "Don't Look Here If You're Seeking Susan." Review of *Swimming in a Sea of Death: A Son's Memoir,* by David Rieff. *The Observer,* June 15, 2008. http://www.guardian.co.uk/books/jun/15/biography.features7.html.

Matuschka. "The Body Beautiful." *MAMM,* Sept.–Oct. 2008. http://www.mamm.com/highlights.

Matuschka. "Why I Did It." *Glamour,* Sept. 1993. http://www.songster.net/projects/matuschka/why.html.

McCloud, Scott. *Understanding Comics: The Invisible Art.* New York: HarperCollins, 1998.

McCormick, Sabrina. *No Family History: The Environmental Links to Breast Cancer.* New York: Rowman and Littlefield, 2009.

McCreery, Allison. "Q & A with David Jay of the SCAR Project." *Photographers on*

Photography, March 23, 2011. http://www,popfoto.net/2011/03/23/qa-with-photographer-david-jay-html.

McGuigan, Cathleen. "Annie Leibovitz's Amazing 'Life in Pictures.'" *Newsweek*, Oct. 2, 2006. http://www.msnbc.msn.com/id/14964292/site/newsweek/print/1/displaymode/1098/html.

McKinney, Caitlin. "Leibovitz and Sontag: Picturing an Ethics of Queer Domesticity." *SHIFT: Queen's Journal of Visual and Material Culture* 3 (2010). http://www.shift journal.org/archives/articles/2010/mckinney.

McRobbie, Angela. "While Susan Sontag Lay Dying." *Open Democracy*, Oct. 10, 2006. http://www.opendemocracy.net/people-photography/sontag_3987.jsp.

Metzger, Deena. *Tree*. Culver City, CA: Peace Press, 1978.

Middlebrook, Christina. *Seeing the Crab: A Memoir of Dying before I Do*. New York: Doubleday, 1996.

Miller, Nancy K. "The Posthumous Life of Susan Sontag." In *The Scandal of Susan Sontag*, ed. Barbara Cheng and Jennifer A. Wagner-Lawlor, 205–16. New York: Columbia University Press, 2009.

Mitchell, David T., and Sharon L. Snyder. *Narrative Prosthesis: Disability and the Dependencies of Discourse*. Ann Arbor: University of Michigan Press, 2000.

Mitchell, W. J. T. *Picture Theory: Essays on Verbal and Visual Representation*. Chicago: University of Chicago Press, 1994.

Morris, David M. *Illness and Culture in the Postmodern Age*. Berkeley: University of California Press, 1998.

Mukherjee, Siddhartha. *The Emperor of All Maladies: A Biography of Cancer*. New York: Scribner, 2010.

Mulvey, Laura. "Visual Pleasures and Narrative Cinema." *Screen* 16 (1975): 6–18.

Myers, Art. *Winged Victory: Altered Images Transcending Breast Cancer*. San Diego: Photographic Gallery of Fine Art Books, 1996.

Norton, Meredith. *Lopsided: How Having Breast Cancer Can Be Really Distracting*. New York: Viking, 2008.

Nussbaum, Martha. *Hiding from Humanity: Disgust, Shame, and the Law*. Princeton: Princeton University Press, 2004.

Oliver, Kelly. *Witnessing: Beyond Recognition*. Minneapolis: University of Minnesota Press, 2001.

Olson, James S. *Bathsheba's Breast: Women, Cancer, and History*. Baltimore: Johns Hopkins University Press, 2002.

Orenstein, Peggy. "Moving Beyond Pink Ribbons." *Los Angeles Times*, Feb. 15, 2012. http://articles/latimes.com/2012/feb/15/opinion/la-oe-orenstein-komen-20120215.

Orenstein, Peggy. "The Trouble with These Boobie Bracelets." *Los Angeles Times*, Apr. 19, 2011. http://www.latimes.com/2011/apr19/opinion/la-oe-orenstein-boobies-20110419.

Patterson, Karen. "Race, Genetics and Cancer: Does Ancestry Play a Role in Cancer Risk and Outcome?" *CURE: Cancer Updates, Research and Education (Supplement)*, Winter 2009, 13–17.

Pekar, Harvey, and Joyce Brabner. *Our Cancer Year.* New York: Four Walls Eight Windows, 1994.

Phelan, Peggy. *Mourning Sex: Performing Public Memories.* London: Routledge, 1997.

Picardie, Ruth. *Before I Say Goodbye: Reflections and Observations from One Woman's Final Year.* New York: Henry Holt, 1997.

Plath, Sylvia. "Lady Lazarus." In *Ariel: The Restored Edition,* 14–17. New York: Harper Perennial, 2004.

Pollock, Griselda. "Dying, Seeing, Feeling: Transforming the Ethical Space of Feminist Aesthetics." In *The Life and Death of Images: Ethics and Aesthetics,* ed. Diarmuid Costello and Dominic Willsdon, 213–35. Ithaca: Cornell University Press, 2008.

Pollock, Griselda. "Femininity: Aporia or Sexual Difference?" Introduction to Bracha L. Ettinger, *The Matrixial Borderspace,* 1–38. Minneapolis: University of Minnesota Press, 2006.

Port, Dina Roth. *Previvors: Facing the Breast Cancer Gene and Making Life-Changing Decisions.* New York: Penguin, 2010.

Prijatel, Patricia. "The Chemo Brain Mystery." *MAMM,* Sept.–Oct. 2008. http://www.mamm.com/highlights.

Proctor, Robert N. *Cancer Wars: How Politics Shapes What We Know and Don't Know about Cancer.* New York: Basic Books, 1995.

"Progress and Promise in Breast Cancer 2010." *CURE: Cancer Updates, Research & Education (Supplement),* Winter 2010.

Queller, Jessica. *Pretty Is What Changes: Impossible Choices, the Breast Cancer Gene, and How I Defied My Destiny.* New York: Spiegel and Grau, 2008.

Rabin, Roni Caryn. "Study Finds Rise in Choice of Double Mastectomies." *New York Times,* Oct. 23, 2007. http://www.nytimes.com/2007/10/23/health/23breast.html.

Rabinovitch, Dina. *Take Off Your Party Dress: When Life's Too Busy for Breast Cancer.* London: Pocket Books, 2007.

Rawson, Mary. *Stephanie: A Story of Transformation.* Dir. Charlee Brodsky, 2000. VHS.

Reibstein, Janet. *Staying Alive: A Family Memoir.* New York: Bloomsbury, 2002.

Rich, Adrienne. *Of Woman Born: Motherhood as Experience and Institution.* New York: Bantam Books, 1977.

Rieff, David. "Illness as More Than Metaphor." *New York Times Magazine,* Dec. 4, 2005. http://www.nytimes.com/2005/12/04/magazine/04sontag.html.

Rieff, David. *Swimming in a Sea of Death: A Son's Memoir.* New York: Simon and Schuster, 2008.

Roiphe, Katie. "Without Metaphor." Review of *Swimming in a Sea of Death: A Son's Memoir,* by David Rieff. *New York Times Book Review,* Feb. 3, 2008, 11.

Romm, Robin. *The Mercy Papers: A Memoir of Three Weeks.* New York: Simon and Schuster, 2009.

Rudnick, Joanna. *In the Family.* First-Run Features, 2008. DVD.

Rugg, Linda Haverty. *Picturing Ourselves: Photography and Autobiography.* Chicago: University of Chicago Press, 1997.

Saltzman, Lisa. *Making Memory Matter: Strategies of Remembrance in Contemporary Art.* Chicago: University of Chicago Press, 2006.

Sather, Jeanne. "Introducing Breast Cancer Joe." Oct. 30, 2008. http://www.assertive patient.com/cancer_humor.

Schultz, Jane E. "(Un)body Double: A Rhapsody on Hairless Identity." *Literature and Medicine* 28, no. 2 (Fall 2009): 371–93.

Scott, Janny. "From Annie Leibovitz: Life, and Death, Examined." *New York Times,* Oct. 6, 2006. http://www.nytimes.com/2006/10/6/arts/design/06leib.html.

Sedgwick, Eve Kosofsky. *A Dialogue on Love.* Boston: Beacon, 1999.

Sedgwick, Eve Kosofsky. "My Bald Head." *MAMM,* Jan. 2001. http://www.mamm .com/highlights.

Sedgwick, Eve Kosofsky. "White Glasses." In *Tendencies,* 252–66. Durham: Duke University Press, 1999.

Silver, Marc. "Cancer Heroes: Six Cancer Survivors Share Their Stories and Their Missions." *CURE: Cancer Updates, Research and Education (Supplement),* Winter 2009, 19–25.

Silverman, Kaja. *The Threshold of the Visible World.* New York: Routledge, 1996.

Singer, Natasha. "In Breast Reconstruction, Some Hidden Choices." *New York Times,* Dec. 23, 2008, A1, A17.

Smith, Roberta. "Photographer to the Stars, With an Earthbound Side." Review of "A Photographer's Life, 1990–2005." Exhibition by Annie Leibovitz, Brooklyn Museum. *New York Times,* Oct. 20, 2006. http:// www.nytimes.com/2006/10/20/arts/ design/20anni.html.

Smith, Sidonie. "Identity's Body." In *Autobiography and Postmodernism,* ed. Kathleen Ashley, Leigh Gilmore, and Gerald Peters, 266–92. Amherst: University of Massachusetts Press, 1994.

Smith, Sidonie, and Julia Watson. "Introduction: Mapping Women's Self-Representation at Visual/Textual Interfaces." In *Interfaces: Women/Autobiography/ Image/Performance,* ed. Sidonie Smith and Julia Watson, 1–46. Ann Arbor: University of Michigan Press, 2002.

Smith, Sidonie, and Julia Watson. *Reading Autobiography: A Guide for Interpreting Life Narratives.* Minneapolis: University of Minnesota Press, 2001.

Somerstein, Rachel. "American Masters: Annie Leibovitz." *www.pbs.org,* June 2008. http://www.pbs.org/wnet/americanmasters/database/leibovitz_a.html.

Sontag, Susan. *As Consciousness Is Harnessed to Flesh: Journals and Notebooks, 1964– 1980.* Ed. David Rieff. New York: Farrar, Straus and Giroux, 2012.

Sontag, Susan. *Illness as Metaphor.* New York: Farrar, Straus and Giroux, 1977.

Sontag, Susan. *On Photography.* New York: Dell, 1977.

Sontag, Susan. *Regarding the Pain of Others.* New York: Farrar, Straus and Giroux, 2003.

Sontag, Susan. "Regarding the Torture of Others." *New York Times Magazine,* May 23, 2004. http://www.nytimes.com/2004/05/23/magazine/23PRISONS.html.

Spence, Jo. *Cultural Sniping: The Art of Transgression.* London: Routledge, 1995.

Spence, Jo. "Marked Up for Amputation" and "Property of Jo Spence?" *Jo Spence Memorial Archive.* http://www.hosted.aware.easynet.co.uk/jospence/jo1.htm.

Spence, Jo. *Putting Myself in the Picture: A Political, Personal and Photographic Autobiography.* Seattle: Real Comet Press, 1988.

Springen, Karen. "No Guarantees." *Newsweek,* Aug. 27, 2008. http://www.newsweek .com/2008/8-26/no-guarantees.html.

Stacey, Jackie. *Teratologies: A Cultural Study of Cancer.* London: Routledge, 1997.

Steingraber, Sandra. *Living Downstream: An Ecologist Looks at Cancer and the Environment.* New York: Addison Wesley, 1997.

Stoddard Holmes, Martha. "Cancer Comix: Narrating Cancer through Sequential Art." Conference lecture, *Cancer Stories.* Indiana University/Purdue University at Indianapolis, Oct. 2008.

Stott, Andrew. *Comedy.* New York: Routledge, 2005.

Sulik, Gayle. *Pink Ribbon Blues: How Breast Cancer Culture Undermines Women's Health.* Oxford: Oxford University Press, 2010.

Tanner, Laura E. *Lost Bodies: Inhabiting the Borders of Life and Death.* Ithaca: Cornell University Press, 2006.

Thernstrom, Melanie. *The Pain Chronicles: Cures, Myths, Mysteries, Prayers, Diaries, Brain Scans, Healing, and the Science of Suffering.* New York: Farrar, Straus and Giroux, 2010.

Thomson, David. "Death Kit." Review of *A Photographer's Life, 1990–2005,* by Annie Leibovitz. *New Republic Online,* Feb. 22, 2007. http://www.powells.com/review /2007_02_22.html.

Tuttle, T. M. et al. "Increasing Use of Contralateral Prophylactic Mastectomy for Breast Cancer Patients: A Trend toward More Aggressive Surgical Treatment." *Journal of Clinical Oncology* 25, no. 33 (Nov. 2007): 5203–9.

Van Schaick, Elizabeth. "Palimpsest of Breast: Representation of Breast Cancer in the Work of Deena Metzger and Jo Spence." *Temple University Graduate Magazine,* Fall 1998. http://www.temple.edu/gradmag/fall98/schaick.htm.

Wear, Delese. Review of *The Summer of Her Baldness: A Cancer Improvisation,* by Catherine Lord. *Literature and Medicine* 23, no. 2 (2004): 378–81.

Wexler, Alice. *Mapping Fate: A Memoir of Family, Risk, and Genetic Research.* Berkeley: University of California Press, 1996.

Williams, Christopher Kwesi O., ed. *Breast Cancer in Women of African Descent.* Dordrecht, The Netherlands: Springer, 2006.

Willis, Jack. *Saving Jack: A Man's Struggle with Breast Cancer.* Norman: University of Oklahoma Press, 2009.

Wilson, Annie. Review of "A Photographer's Life, 1990–2005," Exhibition by Annie Leibovitz, Legion of Honor Museum, San Francisco. www.poeticandchic.com, Mar. 1, 2008. http://www.poeticandchic.com/home/2008/3/1/annie-Leibovitz-a-photographers-life-1990-2005.html.

Wisenberg, S. L. *The Adventures of Cancer Bitch.* Iowa City: University of Iowa Press, 2009.

Wisenberg, S. L. "Bitching and Blogging through Breast Cancer." *Northwestern,* Summer 2010: 20–21.

Yalom, Marilyn. *A History of the Breast.* New York: Ballantine Books, 1997.

Zuger, Abigail. "A Fight for Life Consumes Both Mother and Son." Review of *Swimming in A Sea of Death: A Son's Memoir,* by David Rieff. *New York Times.* Jan. 29, 2008. http://www.nytimes.com/2008/01/29/health/29book.html.

Index